bag lady: A Memoir

Also by Sandra Benítez

A Place Where the Sea Remembers
Bitter Grounds
The Weight of All Things
Night of the Radishes

bag lady

A MEMOIR

A triumphant true story of loss, illness and recovery

For Betty,

by

Sandra Benítez

May your own true stories restore and preserve you.

Paz...

Sandra Benitez

Benítez Books
Edina, Minnesota
www.sandrabenitez.com

Printed in the United States of America.

Benítez, Sandra

bag lady: A Memoir / Sandra Benítez 1st edition

ISBN: 0-9774848-0-7

1. Ileostomy — Memoir 2. Inflammatory Bowel Disease
3. Ulcerative Colitis 4. Twins 5. Alcoholism
6. Hispanic American Women 7. Creative Writing

SAN 257-7097

Cover photograph: Ed Bock Photography, Minneapolis, MN
Book and cover design: Paul Deák, Minneapolis, MN
Copy editing: Nickie Dillon, Minneapolis, MN

This book is for Anita Marina Ables de Alvarez, the sister whose life and presence has more than made up for the twin sister I lost. And in loving memory of our parents, James Quentin Ables and Martha Benítez de Ables.

ACKNOWLEDGMENTS

My profound thanks to my husband, Jim Kondrick, whose love and support kept me going throughout much of my illness and during all of my recovery. In equal measure to my sons, Christopher Title and Jon Title, who never turned away when I needed them.

My gratitude goes to my doctors, Dr. Robert D. Mackie, Minnesota Gastroenterology, Minneapolis, MN; Dr. Robert D. Madoff, Chief, Division of Colon and Rectal Surgery, University of Minnesota; and Dr. Carlos Emilio Alvarez, colon and rectal surgeon, Miami, FL. Thanks, as well, to Jodi Buehring, Dr. Mackie's then nurse practitioner. Gracias, gracias to nurse Susie, my enterostomal therapist, whose last name I never wrote down, I'm sorry to admit, but whose dedication and compassion make her a paragon of her profession. These men and women helped me to be the healthy, happy individual I am today.

To Faith Sullivan, never-ending hugs for enabling the Big Connection.

As always, gracias del corazón a el Espiritu Santo and to la Virgen Milagrosa. Unseen, but ever present.

TO THE READER

This is a book about my thirty-year struggle with inflammatory bowel disease, and my liberation from this tyrannical master through radical surgery. Ultimately, it is about the new life I've come to live after surgery. What this book does *not* contain is an explanation and discussion of inflammatory bowel disease, its various treatments, methods of surgery, and the myriad of products and appliances that can be used after surgery. There are a number of such books covering these topics and I provide the titles of a few of them in the list of resources at the end.

As with all personal stories, mine is a unique account and is meant only to shed a light on one journey, *my* journey, and not to be interpreted as *the way.* The stories contained here are peppered with names of body parts and words usually skirted in polite conversation. These unmentionables accompany a function even more basic than sex, and so it's a dilemma to write about something most people hesitate to talk about. But I'll forge ahead, because I believe it is essential to bring out of the shadows a topic as serious as inflammatory bowel disease and all that it can lead to: colon cancer, topping the list.

My hope in writing this book is to make the general population aware of a disease most sufferers keep hidden, but most important, to give support and encouragement to those who are on the brink of surgery and to those who have undergone it and have doubts about the future.

In addition, the information and stories contained here are meant to help the families and friends of patients understand their loved ones' reality.

To all, I repeat the refrain from a popular tune, but with my own twist:

Try not to worry. Try to be happy.

Paz,

Sandra Benítez
Edina, Minnesota
October, 2005

The patient has to start by treating illness not as a disaster, but as a narrative, a story. Stories are antibodies against illness and pain.

— Anatole Broyard

INTRODUCTION
by Jane E. Brody

FEW IF ANY OF US get through life without having to endure a significant burden, but for some the burdens are more serious or more numerous than for others. Sandra Benítez is among the latter. But in reading *bag lady,* the memoir of her most extraordinary and interesting life and how she managed to weather the trial life threw to her, you cannot help but revel in the humor and joie de vivre with which she approached the many obstacles to happiness that have been thrown in her path during her 60-plus years.

Sandy, as she is called by family and friends, is a true survivor, a resilient, resourceful, talented and amusing person who had to learn over and over again how to turn a sow's ear into a silk purse. Reading her memoir is truly inspiring, and can prove helpful, not just to people faced with similar medical problems, but to anyone who has to cope with a serious challenge to comfort, convenience and personal fulfillment.

The very title of this volume—"bag lady"—speaks

volumes about the kind of person Sandy is: honest with herself and her readers and more than willing to see the humor in what most would consider a rather unpleasant necessity—having to eliminate bodily wastes into a bag for the rest of one's life after uncontrollable disease necessitates the removal of the entire colon and rectum.

Sandy was plagued for 30 years by a bowel that simply refused to behave in anything like a normal way, no matter how carefully she tried to treat it. The pain, the embarrassment, the time and energy lost to illness, the career and family challenges that her diseased bowel foisted upon her eventually left her with no choice but to get rid of it for good. She is by no means alone. Some 2,000,000 people in the United States suffer from inflammatory bowel disease, a great part of these from ulcerative colitis, a chronic disease in which the large intestine and sometimes also the rectum become inflamed and ulcerated, leading to periodic bouts of bloody diarrhea, abdominal cramps and fever. Millions more have a condition with similar symptoms called Crohn's disease, a chronic inflammation of the intestinal wall that can affect any part of the digestive tract.

The cause or causes of these inflammatory bowel diseases are not known. Nor is there a real cure, although as Sandy Benítez so well documents, when all else fails, for ulcerative colitis, getting rid of the diseased organ provides complete and lasting relief from all symptoms. Best of all, having the surgery eliminates the very real possibility of colon cancer.

This memoir "of loss, illness and recovery," as Sandy Benítez calls it, should be just the remedy needed by those who no longer have a choice but to follow the path she had to brave. Rather than treating her surgery and subsequent dependence upon a "bag" for the rest of her life as a calamity, she found it to be an opportunity—a chance to devote her energies and most agreeable personality to what she loves most, her family, her friends and her writing, and a chance to convey to the many people with inflammatory bowel disease and their families that this is by no means an obstacle to a very happy and successful life.

We could all benefit from an injection of Sandy's attitude and outlook.

Jane E. Brody
Personal Health columnist
The New York Times
August 2005

PREFACE

STORIES: SOMETHING HAPPENING. Something important happening to somebody. A simple formula for a monumental truth: We are all enthralled by story. It's why we converse. Why we gossip. It's why we read. To find out what's happening to others. To learn if what's happening to others might help with what's happening to us.

This is the story of important things happening to me. But mostly, it's the story of how I became a bag lady. Not the usual kind of bag lady, but one who, because of illness and then surgery, wears a bag attached to her belly. It's also the story of all the other women who I am: daughter, sister, wife, mother, grandmother, friend. Writer, too, because being a writer allows me to examine and reflect upon all the selves who've made me me.

Though this is a tale about me and my bag, it is not a unique tale. If you think about it, in one way or another, we are all bag people with stories to tell. Each of us totes a bag of our own, be it evident or not: loss of a loved one, a career gone nowhere, addiction, bankruptcy, tragedies and heavy sorrows of whatever ilk. How easy the toting depends on our acknowledging our baggage's presence, on our desire to accept and embrace it, on our ability to unload it (as in unburdening, as in letting go), and finally, on our commitment to taking care of ourselves, baggage and all, as we stride through this world.

Following these simple rules, it's how I make the best of my bag situation.

BEFORE SURGERY

AS THE SAYING GOES, pictures don't lie. The photo I was studying looked like someone had opened a package of raw hamburger and poked a finger through it: a tube of angry red meat grimacing up at me. It was October 1994 and I was propped up on a bed at Abbott Northwestern Hospital, in Minneapolis, still shaky and perspiring from the colonoscopy I'd endured. The pain in my gut and in my butt was so severe I whimpered to my husband, "Just shoot me, Jim. Put me down like a dog."

My surgeon, Dr. Robert Madoff, also stood next to the bed. He had provided the photo. A souvenir straight off the colonoscopy monitor screen.

"This is bad," I said, for it was not hamburger I was looking at. It was the inside of my colon.

Dr. Madoff nodded. "It's not good."

Jim took the photo from my hand, gulping as he gazed at it. He turned to look at me. "I think it's time, Sandy."

"Yeah, it might well be." I allowed myself to go limp

against the pillows. Maybe it was time. Time for TBS, The Big Surgery. Time to say goodbye, adios, sayonara to this diseased part of me that was wreaking havoc with my body, with my life.

The surgery that was being strongly recommended by Dr. Madoff, by Dr. Bob Mackie, my gastroenterologist, by Dr. Carlos Emilio Alvarez, my brother-in-law and a colon and rectal surgeon in Miami, is called a total proctocolectomy with ileostomy. The first two words are the name for a procedure that removes colon, rectum and anus. To be sure, body areas with little cachet, but hey, we were talking about *my* body's areas here. Funny how precious these ignoble body parts become when the prospect of losing them looms.

Though I'd been ill for almost thirty years with ulcerative colitis, though each year the risk of colon cancer grew alarmingly, a decision to have such radical surgery was not an easy one. It meant my backside would be sewn shut; it meant having a permanent ileostomy, which would result in my living with a bag for the rest of my life. I was 53. The long years ahead with a bag hanging from my side stretched out before me like the Alcan Highway.

I had no idea what a bag looked like. I had no idea how it would be attached. How daily elimination could be accomplished. I had no idea what the surgery entailed. I guess I could have looked it up, but this I had not done. Maybe because it would have seemed like a self-fulfilling prophecy. God knows I'd researched and studied everything else about what ailed me. I was up on symptoms, complications, treatments, medications, side-effects. Each time I stepped into Bob Mackie's office, I worried that he'd tire of my incessant questions. But thankfully, he isn't that kind of human being. Over the years that he treated me, he took his time, making me feel as if I were his only patient. My brother-in-law was equally helpful. Sometimes it was the middle of the night when I'd call him in Miami. I'd be in pain and bleeding, weak as boiled linguini and out of my mind from the heavy doses of steroids I had to take, yet Carlos Emilio was at all times patient, understanding and kind. But more and more, he'd been urging me to end my misery and have the surgery. "Once you do it, you'll wonder why you waited so long," he often said.

Dr. Madoff said it now, adding, "You won't believe how good you'll feel after it's over."

I turned to Jim. "What do you think?"

"I think you should do it, babe."

I let out a long breath. The breath I'd been holding for such a long time. "Okay. What the hell, let's go for it."

"Good decision," Madoff said. "You won't regret it."

• • •

It was late Monday, and the surgery was scheduled for Thursday. I'd have two days in which the doctors would try to ameliorate this latest flare-up that had landed me in the hospital for the umpteenth time, two days to be prepped for the surgery that would change my life—maybe even save it—given that colon cancer was a real and constant threat.

Enter nurse Susie, the ET or the enterostomal therapist. Her ash blond hair flipped up at the ends. Her freckled face featured a toothy smile. "Doris Day-perky" came readily to mind. It was she who would bring me up to date on her specialty, on a world that included the words *ileum, stoma, appliance* (appliance?), *adhesive, film barrier, clip.*

Susie gave me the lowdown on the surgery. In my case, a two-part procedure. First, there was the *abdomino-perineal resection,* in which two openings would be made: one through the abdomen, the other down along the perineum, the area behind the genitals to the anus. Through the former, Madoff would remove the entirety of the colon or large intestine, through the latter, the rectum and anus.

Once free of the diseased tissue, he would perform an *ileostomy,* a surgically created opening through the right side of my stomach. To do this, he would bring the *ileum,* the end of the small intestine, up through the abdominal wall to form a *stoma* through which body waste would flow into a bag, or *appliance.*

A more common procedure is the *colostomy*, in which the surgical opening is usually made on the left side of the stomach, and which involves bringing a section of colon up through the skin. This, however, was impossible in my case, given that my colon was being removed entirely.

Susie gave me this quick sketch of my surgery, for which I was thankful, but in truth I did not let my mind rest on any of it. On Thursday, I'd allow myself to be anesthetized and let Madoff do his thing. Afterward, I'd cope with whatever was presented me.

Still, there were matters that needed my attention. To wit, Susie asked, "Have you ever seen a stoma?"

"Can't say I have." Susie was holding something behind her back. A surprise?

"Okay, I'm going to show you a model of one right now, but I don't want you to be shocked. A stoma is very red." She drew her hand in sight, then opened it before me.

I let out a small yip. Lying on her palm was a bright red plug as long and thick as the end of my thumb.

"This is what it looks like. 'Stoma' is from the Greek and means 'mouth.' Think of it as a little faucet. Your surgeon will pull it through the opening in your right side, turn it inside-out like you do when you cuff a sock, and then sew the edge of it to your tummy to keep it in place. Your stoma will always be red and glistening because it's really your intestinal wall you're seeing."

I took the stoma from her. It was a short red cylinder with a little pucker at the top.

"There's an opening at the top; poke your finger in."

Tentatively, I did. The opening gave and my finger slipped right in. It felt very, very weird.

"A real stoma is moist. Think of the inside of your mouth. The best part is that it has no nerve endings, so that it's completely insensitive to the touch."

Now there was fabulous news.

"So, what's going to happen is that you'll have a stoma protruding from the right side of your tummy. Waste matter will flow from it. Just like from a faucet. And that's where the bag comes in." She produced one for me then: two panels of heavy-gauge, see-through plastic. The bag looked like a huge key hole, round on top and tapering down into a long rectangle of a tail, a tail with an open end. I turned the bag over to see a quarter-size hole in the middle of the top of the bag. This opening was surrounded by a circle of rubbery material that felt tacky to the touch.

"What you're feeling is adhesive," she said. "Picture your stoma poking out of your side, then picture your stoma slipping right into that hole. That sticky circle will then lie against your stomach and stick to it. That's why it's often called an 'appliance,' because it's 'applied' to your skin."

"But will it stay stuck?"

"It will. For now, all you need to know is that when you come out of surgery, your bag will already be in place. Your stoma will start working soon after you start eating and waste is produced."

After you start eating. How long had it been since I'd had a real meal? For months and months my menu had consisted of consommé and Jell-O and sometimes, for a treat, a piece of Melba toast.

Susie continued, "Waste will flow from your stoma and be caught in the bag."

"But the bag has an opening at the end." I pulled the two panels apart at the tail to show her.

"You'll use a clip to seal the end."

I nodded, as if I understood. I was lying in bed, so many questions still swirling in my head. How long would I be wearing each bag? Did I have to put on a new one every time I emptied? And what exactly would I empty? Would it be the same as poop? Suddenly, it all seemed too much to take in. I asked myself, Could I do this? Did I even want to do this? I could, if I wanted, have put the brakes on the plans. I could tell the surgeon, the gastro man, my brother-in-law, that, for now, I was going to pass on surgery. That for now I was going to stay in the hospital until the flare-up subsided and then I'd go back home to continue with the cramping and the bleeding and the nausea and the bloating. That I'd continue taking the prednisone that made me crazy, that caused my eyes to blur, that caused my face to go round as a pumpkin, my cheeks to sprout fuzz, that brought on bouts of joint-pain in my hands and feet, pain so severe in my feet that sometimes to get around I had to crawl across the floor. I'd tell them that I liked the daily doses of 6-MP, the immunosuppressive drug that caused my blood counts to go so low I was often so weak and tired I had trouble getting up. I'd tell them I didn't at all mind the painful iron injections I often needed to bring my blood-counts up. Injections of serum so thick and dark that my buttocks looked like I'd been thwacked with two-by-fours. I'd tell them I really didn't mind taking the nightly doses of mineral oil to help keep me from straining as I sat, for hours and hours, on the toilet. That it was no big deal that, sometimes, when I was off the toilet, the need to defecate came on so strongly, that no matter how much I hurried, the toilet was never near enough. And I'd tell them that it was no biggie, no biggie at all, that on that one particular time, when I was in the grocery store parking lot, lifting up the trunk lid, my personal bottom-gates loosened and out it came, poop and mucous and that sweet sickly smell, it all slipping down my legs and into my shoes. I could, if I wanted, tell my doctors that I'd just as soon continue living this life of misery. This life, that for a long time, didn't seem like a life at all.

"You know what?" I said to nurse Susie. "I'm totally exhausted."

"Right. You need to get some rest. Let these IV fluids make you better."

What was dripping out of those IV bags and into my skinny arms was glucose and potassium and prednisone and who knows what other medical concoction. I just wanted to float on the raft that was my bed, maybe float away into oblivion.

"One thing, though, before you nod off. I'm going to adhere this bag to your tummy. That way, you can start getting the feel of an appliance at your side."

"Go for it."

She lifted my gown and there my poor body lay, breasts sliding limply off to the sides, stomach a concave hollow, hip bones poking up pathetically. My legs were so thin, the thighs could be completely encircled by a pair of hands.

"There you go," Susie said. And there it was. The bag applied to my right side and sitting somewhat askance so that its long tail obscured my pubic bone.

She gave the bag a little pat. Pulled down my gown. Pulled up the sheet and coverlet. "You get some rest now. I'll be back tomorrow."

I laid my hands over my tummy, experiencing for the first time the unfamiliar feel of plastic against flesh.

• • •

The next day, the day before surgery, soon after lunch, Jim came to spend time with me. He patiently listened to me go round and round about whether I should cancel the surgery or not. I'd been wearing the test bag for a day and a half, with nurse Susie adhering it to one spot, and then soon after, moving it to another place just inches away. When I questioned what she was doing, she assured me that proper bag placement was critical to comfortable bag-wearing later. Where the bag sat, and where the tail rested, were very important. Choosing the stoma site would determine this, and to this end, she'd poked and prodded my belly, examining it closely as I stood, as I sat and bent at the waist, looking for areas where the flesh would fold or crease, thus making it difficult for stoma protrusion and bag adhesion. Late yesterday, in fact, she'd selected my "sweet spot": three inches to the right of my bellybutton and one inch down from that. She'd made a big X on my skin with black ink. Later today, she would return to "tattoo" the spot with permanent ink, a necessary detail so that Madoff would know precisely where to construct the stoma opening. I didn't want to think about all of that. In fact, I was allowing hospital preparations to continue, while still holding out the possibility that I could pull the plug on the whole shebang. It gave me comfort to do this. It allowed me to think I had a modicum of control over events that were coming at me like a steamroller.

Sitting up in bed, my lunch tray holding plates of soft food I'd only picked at—Malto-Meal, scrambled eggs, toast, Gatorade—a feeling of pure panic washed over me. A sourness rose up in my throat, and I threw a hand over my mouth for fear that I'd vomit. So, too, the need to use the toilet assailed me so fiercely that I scrambled to throw off the bed sheet. Jim, noting my wild eyes and being so familiar with these bouts, helped me to my feet and held me up until I made it into the bathroom.

"I'll be right here," he said, when he closed the door.

I swallowed down the acridness in my throat, fumbling with the ties of my hospital gown. I could not stand anything against my flesh. The panic I felt caused my skin to go instantly hot. I felt the sweat dotting my upper lip. Felt it breaking along my brow. I threw my gown off, but left the bag on because I had to. I sat on the pot and out of me poured razor blades. I bit my lip to keep from crying out, but I could not help the moans I emitted, deep and low and otherworldly. I was in the bathroom for almost an hour. When I got up from the seat, the toilet bowl was bright red. The room was sweetly foul. The particular odor of my condition.

I slipped on my gown again and cracked the door to try to keep the smell in, and through the opening I saw Jim. He sat in the chair beside the bed, his head in his hands, his shoulders heaving.

I shuffled over to him and he jumped up and helped me into bed, his face wet with tears. "You've got to do something, babe. You can't go on like this."

"I know, Jaimsey. I know."

We had a little talk. He would go home and fetch my tall votive candle of the Miraculous Virgin Mary. He would fetch my incense holder and a stick of copal incense. These items I lighted every morning when I readied myself to write. Today, I'd light them in a hospital bathroom. I'd sit on the throne and say a long goodbye to body parts that had served me as best they could, but that were now surely dying.

• • •

Much later, after Susie had come in and pricked my belly with a needle at X-marks-the-spot, after she colored the incision with green dye, after I'd had a soothing sitz bath, and then a shower, I sprinkled myself with baby powder, just like I used to sprinkle my babies after their baths. I donned a clean gown and slipped into the bathroom.

I don't know. A person might have trouble understanding someone like me: a person who believes in the power of rituals. Prayer. Meditation. Candle lighting and incense burning.

But a ritual for a colon? For a rectum and an anus? Come on, already, you might say. But all I can tell you is, hey, it works for me. It works for me because in ritualizing something as significant as bidding Godspeed to whatever it is we find necessary to surrender, we acknowledge the leave-taking and can perhaps start to practice acceptance.

A noble thing, acceptance. A noble thing to strive for.

And so it was that I lit the candle and the incense wand, that I switched off the light and sat on the closed lid of the pot in my birthday suit, the room glowing goldenly, the pungency of copal filling the space. I breathed the scent in deeply and spread a hand over my tummy incised with a green X and applied with a bag. I reached around with the other hand and cupped my bottom tenderly.

Adios, I murmured. Adios, which in Spanish means "to God." I give back to God what He has blessed me with. Gracias, I added. Gracias dear parts of me, gracias for your long and hard labor at absorbing, storing and eliminating. Praised be, I continued, praised be a new day without pain, without agony. Welcome, I concluded. Welcome little bag. Welcome little faucet. Little spout.

I sat there like that, holding on to myself while the tears came and the fear rose up and I allowed it in and gave it its due until it subsided.

• • •

The Big Surgery day, and I was the star of the production. The operating room was filled with blue-robed and white-masked people. Dr. Madoff was ready to roll. He had selected, he said, beautiful calming tunes to play on the CD as he worked. Helga, the surgical nurse chosen especially by my stepdaughter, Denise, a surgical nurse at Abbott herself, had been soothing and assuring me all the way down from my room. She stood next to the anesthetist, who smiled behind his mask. I could see the smile in his eyes. “How about it?” he asked. “Shall we get this show on the road?”

There was a big clock on the wall across from where I lay. It was mid-afternoon. When I wake up, I thought, I’ll be a bag lady. I gave Helga and the anesthetist a thumbs up. Helga squeezed my hand. “Don’t you worry about a thing.”

“Okay,” I said, and closed my eyes, soon tunneling way, way back into the shimmering whiteness that contained all my stories.

MY LIFE AS A BAG LADY started long before I began to wear my little bag. It began with stomachaches and straining and long sessions on the pot. Over time, these maladies escalated to inflammatory bowel syndrome (IBS), which finally erupted forty years ago into inflammatory bowel disease (IBD): in my case, ulcerative colitis (UC). Crohn's disease is yet another form of IBD. Over the years, the search for the cause of UC and its treatment have undergone radical changes, but in a medical dictionary of symptoms I possess, a book published in 1967, under "ulcerative colitis" comes a description that paints it as an ulcerous inflammation of the large intestine. It goes on to say that UC can manifest itself as a weak spot in some "unusual personalities." That more women than men suffer it. That sometimes an emotional upset can set off an acute phase. Oooo, interesting. I remember reading the description, over and over, trying hard to ascertain the unusualness in my personality that would cause a weakness in my gut, a weakness that, over time, had brought on a tide of symptoms, going from the pesky to the downright nightmarish.

Every family has its totem stories, that is, particular stories that we ascribe to one another and that help identify each member's unique idiosyncrasies and talents. She's the shy one. He's the creative one. Don't rile her, she'll bite. Put a nickel in, and he'll talk your ear off. These identifiers and the remember-when stories that surround them make for hilarity and good-natured ribbing at big family gatherings, but they have their negative effect as well, because generally, they mark people with labels from which they rarely can escape. If they do seek a transformation, it's accomplished with great difficulty, most always against much family resistance.

In my family, I was the sensitive one. At the slightest hint of fault or trouble—frustration, sorrow, anger, fear—mine or anyone else's, my stomach churned and my mouth found my thumb.

Perhaps this sensitivity really began when Susana, my identical twin sister, passed away thirty-seven days after our birth. Maybe as I lay in the little boat of my Isolette placed right next to hers, that ineffable bond that connected us gave a tug as her essence went rising up. Up, up like a sigh. One moment there, the next gone. Then tiny Sandra, left behind to go it alone.

Maybe my perfectionism started then, as well. Because over time, I've come to understand that Susana's shadow has been my constant companion, even if I was aware of it or not. Since her death I'd striven to make up for her departure by being perfect, both for my mother's benefit and for my own. In so doing, I've lived my own life while attempting to live the life my sister never had. Twice good, twice nice, twice perfect. An exhausting endeavor in a world where perfection should be left only to God.

• • •

I was diagnosed with ulcerative colitis in 1972, when I was thirty-one, but I'd been ailing for years before that.

Although born in Washington, D.C., I grew up in Latin America. My father, James Quentin Ables, a Missouri farm-boy, had, after his military service, moved to the capital to work as a Senate page. In Washington, he had fallen in love with Martha Benítez, a Puerto Rican beauty. My mother opened my father's eyes to the foreign and exotic. So it wasn't any surprise that, after their wedding, Daddy signed up with the Foreign Service. This decision must have been a bittersweet one: the job would distance them from the grief they experienced when Susana died, but having to leave her behind in a Maryland cemetery was heartbreaking. To Mami it must have been tantamount to abandonment.

I was just over a year old when our small family moved to Mexico City, where Daddy served as Vice-Consul, Military and Agricultural Attaché at the American embassy. Nine months later, my sister Anita made her appearance, smack in the middle of an earthquake. Four years after the happy shake-up, our traveling resumed. Daddy was transferred to El Salvador and assumed the same position he'd held before. At long last, we were able to settle down. We stayed, for a very long time, in what was then a pacific, idyllic little country.

In the late '40s, when I was seven and eight and nine, we lived in the capital, San Salvador, in a house built at the edge of the city, at a place called La Ceiba, named after an imposing silk-cotton tree perched atop its highest hillock. At the embassy, Daddy had been poking through some old files in his office and had chanced across a deed signed by General Maximiliano Martínez, a former president of El Salvador. Martínez was the despot who put down the campesino rebellion in 1932 during which 30,000 Nahuat Indians were massacred. The deed ceded a parcel of land to the United States government in gratitude for something or other.

His curiosity piqued, Daddy, along with Mami, used the embassy's black Ford sedan with its little American flag affixed to the left antenna and drove out to take a look at the property. The U.S. had built an agricultural experimental station there, but the operation had eventually shut down and moved farther out of town. The grounds were expansive: acres of lawns and shrubs, an array of pine, mango and avocado trees, plus circular beds of day lilies, margaritas and hydrangeas. Purple bougainvillea climbed and flourished against whatever surface it ventured toward. Carmine poinsettias grew in tall thickets to form natural fences between the estate and the road. All the vegetation was wildly overgrown when my parents arrived at the place that branched off the main highway at kilometer number six. They turned into the driveway, flanked on both sides by low walls and, shading them, rows of coconut palms, looking like sentinels with feathery headdresses. The driveway was overgrown with weeds so tough and high they rattled the sedan's undercarriage. Up ahead loomed the agricultural station's building: a boxy, stucco edifice sporting a wide overhanging roof and painted the color of mourning doves. Don Tomás, the caretaker, was sitting on the steps when the car clattered in. He ambled over to meet them, his straw hat respectfully at his side. By way of explanation, he pointed to the area. "Ay, Señor," he said, "aquí no hay nada. Se lo llevaron todo." There's nothing here. Everything's been carted off.

Not quite, Daddy had thought. Despite the neglect, possibilities abounded. With the right design, the building might be converted into a proper residence. The floors and the long side-porch were overlaid with dulled and dirty oxblood-colored tiles. But scrubbed and polished, what a grand porch it would be. A sad-looking yard spread out from the porch, but once trimmed and mowed, Mami's dream of living in a country house with spacious grounds, lush with trees and abloom with flowers, seemed about to come true. All that was needed was the ambassador's blessing for restoration and occupancy, and the state department's stamp on the ambassador's approval.

Fortune smiled. Within a month the many triplicated petitions were approved. Within two months, our family was ensconced in paradise. Don Tomás and his wife, Blanca, stayed on—he as the gardener now, she as the "inside girl," which is to say, the cleaning woman. In addition, Mami hired Meches, the laundress, and Adela, the cook. It was 1946. The war was over. We had a country house. Servants. We were flush.

• • •

A year after we moved in, the place resembled a little Eden. The lawn was lush green velvet, the drive graveled, its paralleling walls whitewashed into respectability. A breadfruit tree with spindly branches and palmate leaves grew exotically at the edge of the porch. Next to the house, white and yellow roses formed a long-line bouquet. At mid-yard, cedars gave off their sharp scent. Across the road, the volcán San Salvador towered grandiosely.

One of my favorite spots was at the end of the driveway, where it curved around the back of the house. There, at the edge of the lawn and in the full-brunt of the sun, rose a large flat-topped boulder. Sitting upon its heated surface was soothing to my bottom as well as my tummy, which often pitched a fit. All, it was thought, caused by "something I ate." In Salvador, strange bacteria often came with the food. Because of it, my parents set down a fiat: No street food. But I frequently disobeyed. I loved paletas, popsicles, the orange and lime ones. Both made, most likely, with tainted water. And every now and then, I'd use part of my allowance and treat myself to a small bottle of milk. In Salvador, in the forties, milk was unpasteurized and unhomogenized, but I loved it anyway, and drank it on the sly, most times, before leaving the store. So much more satisfying than the chalky, often lumpy, concoction, made at home with purified water and KLIM (milk spelled backward!), a powdered, yet safe, product. And I loved green mangoes. Pulled off the tree, peeled with my teeth, I devoured them with salt. Like green apples, they were crunchy and tart. Like green apples, they often prompted stomachaches.

Once, when I was eight, I think, I came home from my all-girls Catholic school in my white uniform with the rounded collar and long puffy sleeves. I had on my regimented footwear: black oxfords and long white stockings. My brunette hair was gathered severely into braids and the only concession to color were the red bows dangling at the end. Before going into the house to change, I went to roost on my rock, when Meches, the laundress (I always called her "nana"), came out of the house, her arms laden with just-washed clothing she was about to lay in the sun to bleach. I was sucking my thumb, a habit that comforted me and that no one could break. Of the family, it was only la nana who left me in peace when my thumb plugged up my mouth. No cajoling, no ridiculing, no threats ever came from her.

"¿Qué le pasa?" nana asked. What's the matter?

"Mi cuculito." My little butt. I spoke the words around my thumb. Because she'd inquired, I went on to blurt out what I'd discovered when in the bathtub that morning. I was scrubbing myself and, ¡Ay no!, a tiny bump, back down there, between my buttocks.

Nana nodded and set the clothing down in one sodden heap. "You have to spit on that bump," she said. Being in her fifties, with a wizened face the color of a chestnut, la nana seemed ancient to me. She gathered her salt-and-pepper hair into two skinny braids, the ends of which she tied, day after day, with the same short lengths of frayed purple ribbon.

"Spit on it?" I remember that I couldn't imagine how I might bend back so low that I could accomplish this.

Nana nodded again, this time more vigorously. "You spit on your hand. Like this." She raised a palm to her mouth and pursed her lips and made a wet explosion. "Then you rub your hand over that bump." To demonstrate, she lifted a hip and rubbed, hard it seemed, on the back of her skirt. "You rub and rub. And do it when you first get up, before you have your breakfast."

"How can that be?" Nana was always filled with information, some of which made little sense to me, but which I never ignored. After all, la nana could do magic.

Once, when I lost my baby doll, she'd made four knots in the corner of a handkerchief—to tie up la "anima Juana," who liked to snatch up children's dolls, nana said—and had me place the hankie under my pillow. That evening, shazam!, my baby doll returned to me.

Nana made a puffing sound with her mouth. "¡Hágalo!" she ordered. Do it! She picked up one of Daddy's white shirts and shook it free of wrinkles. Droplets floated in the air, like sparkly rain drops. She went about her business, laying clothing out on the drying patio, my tummy problems quite obviously of no further concern.

And so I did as nana commanded. Every morning, I'd spring out of bed and head for the sunlit bathroom. I'd throw the latch on the door and before I sat on the pot, I'd spit on my hand, ptu!, and slather myself royally. Soon after, the little bump was gone. But the puzzlement of its appearance, the concern it had caused, the miracle of its disappearance, I kept to myself. I was like that. Mundane things I blabbered incessantly about. Deeply personal feelings, I did not voice.

A big mistake when I look back. Perhaps, had I been forthcoming, the tiny terror it evoked might have been assuaged, explained even, by a confession. But I had reasons for keeping silent; I was not the only one in the household with stomach problems. My mother was plagued by them. Once, in a rare moment of self-revelation, Mami told me that when she was a little girl in Puerto Rico, her mother, Abuelita, used to dose her with spoonfuls of charcoal. Mami said, "Mother used to stand there beside me until I got it all down. After, I'd drag a chair over to her dresser and climb up and poke my black tongue out and study it in the mirror."

Later, after Mami's death in 1999, after her absence revealed many things about her, I came to understand how affected my mother had been by the upheaval of her family's relocation from Puerto Rico. Abuelito's, my grandfather's, coffee plantation and his wealth was swept away by a hurricane when Mami was eight. These terrifying winds of change separated the family, for Abuelito had stayed behind as the rest moved, first to New York, and years later, to Washington, D.C., where Susana died. Over the years, Mami rarely mentioned the loss of her child, but it caused her many ailments, the intestinal kind topping the list. These ailments often prompted a change of diet: no beef, no fat, no grains. In fact, at one time and for a few months, her nourishment consisted of meals that looked a lot like baby food. A revelation in and of itself.

Compared to my mother, my complaints were minor. Still, she made sure I received my own remedies: té de manzanilla y galletas María, chamomile tea and arrowroot cookies, which Adela, the cook, had ready when I arrived from school. And if I was specially good, after I had my treat, and while she worked at the ironing board, nana allowed me to sprawl on the cot in the laundry room with my thumb in my mouth. I liked the way she'd touch a finger to her tongue and lay it on the iron's hot plate, one time, two, until there was a satisfying sizzle. As a way to engage her, I'd often ask for a story. "Cuénteme el cuento de la Ziguanaba," I'd say. Tell me the one about la Ziguanaba. At first she would harrumph at the request, but soon she'd fix her gaze across the room as if her story were unfurling like a motion picture on the wall.

"Había un vez," she'd begin. "Once upon a time

there lived a woman who was very beautiful. God gave her children and they were beautiful, too." Enrapt, I'd settle back onto the lone pillow on the cot. This legend was the story of the wailing woman who, driven mad by a man's love, abandoned her children so she could join her lover unencumbered. God punished her for this. "'You have abandoned your sons,' God said, 'when I gave them to you for keeps. As punishment, you will search for them until the end of the world.'"

Nana hung the pressed shirt on a wire hanger. She turned to throw me a dark, fierce look. She said, "At night, when you're in bed, if you listen very carefully, you can hear la Ziguanaba. Along the riverbanks and in the woods, she wails, 'Ay, mis hijos.'" Oh, my children.

I shuddered with delight, thinking I could catch, even in the daylight, the sounds of a mother's grief. "¡Uy, Nana!" I'd say and nana, perhaps softened by her own story, ran the iron back and forth over a length of dampened fabric and soon the room grew more redolent with the fragrance of freshly pressed cotton. She laid the hot cloth over my tummy. Ahhhh! A little slice of heaven.

After a while, but still under the story's spell, I'd gone outside to visit el loro, our emerald parrot. His name was Roberto and he spent the day swaying back and forth on his perch, which sat in the shade of one of the mango trees. Roberto's wings were clipped and he was old and so his flying days were over. He accepted patiently his lot as my pet. Sometimes, he'd let me cradle him and he'd mold himself in the half circle of my arm, his tail feathers stiff and quivering. That day, I'd raised a finger to him and he'd blinked his papaya-seed eyes and given me a squawk.

I blinked back and squawked a promise to him, "You are my baby. I would never abandon you."

• • •

Frequently, I did my homework on the porch. Adela always offered a snack: most times cookies, but for a special treat a square of pan dulce, sweet bread, and a glass of fresco de Quaker, a refreshment she made by soaking oatmeal flakes in water and pressing the mash through a sieve. She mixed in icy milk, sweetened it, then whipped the concoction into a froth. I loved the porch and its blood-red tiles. When I sat there, the sun was low and the front yard and the mountain beyond were bathed in yellow-red light. The afternoon smelled delicious: as if all the scents the day had taken up were now floating down.

Chicha, our brown dachshund, liked to keep me company. I'd break off a corner of my treat and share it with her. Chicha's belly was swollen with pups. "Ya va ser," I said to her, parroting what Mami always said. It'll be soon.

At school we were learning the multiplication tables and I found them tiresome and complicated. I much preferred the reading and the writing. Sprawled upon one of the wicker lounge chairs on the porch, a book propped against my thighs, the stories I read transported me to Araby where I, too, could rub a magic lamp, or to a wide white-sand beach where I'd ride like the wind upon the back of a sleek black stallion. I wrote pretend letters. To Ali Baba, to the Princess after she'd tossed uncomfortably upon her mattresses set upon one single pea, to Nancy Drew, proposing a new solution to a mystery she had solved.

Often, as I read or wrote, the servants would pause to observe me as they went from one task to another, and I'd lift my head and see in their eyes an expression that often puzzled me: Wistfulness? Sadness? Envy?

One afternoon, when Adela set my snack down beside me, she asked, "Mi Niña, por favor leáme una carta." My girl, please read a letter for me.

Because of my penchant for all things written, I readily complied. But in some deep part of me, because at almost ten I was capable of doing what she could not, I felt it an obligation. For the most part, however, there was the matter of curiosity. Serving as reader or scribe would provide me a glimpse into someone else's life.

We sat in the kitchen, at the servants' oak table. Scratched and stained and gouged, it rested under the corkscrew staircase leading to their room. A letter had come from Chalatenango, Adela's home. On the onion-skin envelope, the cook's full name (Adela Maria Alvarenga), our address (La Ceiba, Kilometro Número 6, San Salvador), was written in pencil and by a heavy hand, most certainly that of a hired scribe. I slipped the letter out, the paper as thin as the envelope. "Vaya pues," I said, "empezemos." Okay, let's begin.

Adela sat ramrod straight as I began to read. "My dearest sister. I hope that when you receive this you are well of health. We are well of health here, though the weather is chilly and your little Marito has a cold. But don't worry about your boy. Yesterday, I carried him to the healer and he prescribed three drops of ocote oil on a sugar cube. You know how Marito likes his sugar, but he balks at the taste and smell of pine resin, and who can blame the child for that? But don't you worry. I managed to make him take it, though he bawled the whole time. Do you think you could send a few extra colones? We need more of don Pedro's remedy and it costs more than I have. Okay, then, this is all the news. I take my leave for now, hoping that you can forward me what I need so the boy can be well. I hope you are not working too hard there in the capital. I hope you remember to send the money. From the one who loves you and who never forgets you, Your loving sister, Delia María Alvarenga. Oh, and remember, don't worry about the boy."

Message delivered, my young heart brimmed with borrowed anxiousness. Adela had not moved in her chair. Her gaze was set on her opened hands, lying inertly in her lap. Helpless, I said, "Ay, no se aflija," repeating her sister's thrice stated request. Ignoring what else to do, I folded the letter at the crease, slipped it back into its envelope, slid it back across the table.

Had I had an Arabian genie's powers, I would have blown a mental kiss over the letter and transformed the story into an ordinary one. "My dearest sister," I would have read. "I hope that when you receive this you are well of health. We are well of health, too. Your Marito is a robust and happy boy. Though you know how chilly this northern country is, for a good time the weather has been uncommonly warm. Marito plays in the sun, his laughter always a blessing. Next month, when you send money home, can you see your way to including a few extra colones? Your son's shoes needed re-soling, and don Francisco, the cobbler, did the work ahead of time. He said, Pay me when you can. So when you send the extra money, I'll pass it on to him. I hope you are not working too hard there in the capital. I hope you remember the ones who love you, the ones who never do forget you. Your loving sister, Delia María Alvarenga. Oh, and remember, your little boy loves you. He has not forgotten his dearest mother."

As I grew older, I read letters silently to myself, before plunging in. If the situation warranted it, and no harm could come, I'd allow myself the freedom to soften and invent.

I believe it was then that I began to be a fiction writer, though it was thirty-some years later before I gathered the courage to begin.

• • •

Invention. Imagination. Two of the tools of the writer's trade. I used both back then to build a castle in the air. I built it next to the house, at the place where the old foundation of what once might have been an outbuilding (a livery? a workshop?) remained. The space provided me with a unique playground. I dragged in odd pieces of scrap lumber, rolled in big stones and fashioned a table and my own kind of chairs. Around them, in my imagination, I erected walls, setting within these boundaries my first living room, dining room and bedroom, this latter room in the one spot softened by the shade a mango tree provided. In my kitchen, I laid a square of tin over two bricks and, presto!, I had a cooking griddle, just like the one Blanca, don Tomás's wife, had in her cooking shed.

For ideas, I liked to visit don Tomás and Blanca's little one-room house. It rose beyond ours, up at the end of the driveway. The room had a packed-dirt floor, the cooking shed set alongside and leaning into it. A low wall surrounded and defined the place. To beautify it, Blanca set out used lard cans at intervals along the wall. Sprouting from them were red and pink geraniums. One day, when I returned to my imaginary house after school, I found a can with a pink geranium sitting beside the griddle. I ran down the driveway to thank Blanca, and she smiled shyly and shrugged her shoulders. Like Chicha's, her belly was also swollen.

My geranium scented the air with its lemony leaves. As Blanca did, I wished I could build a fire under my own griddle and thereby perfume the air with the added smell of wood smoke. But having matches and making a fire was strictly prohibited. I had to content myself with invention. No matter. I used the bit of masa that Blanca had given me and slapped the dough into a tortilla and laid it on the griddle heated by the sun. I pulled mangoes from my tree and ate them in my kitchen. Green mangoes with salt. Crunchy, tart, delicious.

While I played, nana walked in and out of the laundry room to spread clothing over the bushes so the clothing could whiten in the sun. Watching me, she shook her head and made that little puffing sound she often made in reproof. "Look, Nana," I said. "I'm making dinner." She looked at me with a curious expression. She made her little sound. She said, "What a sight. A rich girl pretending to be poor."

I trailed her into the laundry room, plopped myself down on the cot as she began a new mountain of ironing. Her remark had puzzled me. She'd called me a rich girl, but I was hardly that. Most girls at school were rich: their families owned coffee and cotton plantations; they sailed for Paris and returned with haute couture. At our house, Daddy went to work at the American embassy.

The most important item in Mami's closet was the small strongbox she stashed in a corner, beside her shoes. It was made of gray iron and had a tiny wheel for spinning numbers that, lined up just right, allowed the lid to be raised. The strongbox held a myriad of envelopes, each marked with a household expense and stuffed with colón bills: groceries, rent, laundry, cook, clothing, gardener, inside girl, gifts, entertainment, miscellaneous.

Thinking back upon those times, I remember how Mami often anxiously turned the box's combination dial and lifted its lid. She never said a word, but it was clear to me that sometimes a few envelopes lacked some of their stuffing. This kind of uncertainty caused my tummy to knot up. It placed a worrisome pall over the rest of the day.

Hearing nana's comment back then, I wondered if she were poor. I thought that if I went to her house, I might find out and somehow this would put a light on things. I had to broach the subject obliquely. "Nana, why don't you sleep at our house at night?" She was the only servant who left after work. Juana slept in the laundry room. Don Tomás and Blanca had their little house.

"Because I like to sleep in my own bed."

"Where is your bed?" My pronunciation was a bit garbled because my thumb was resting against the roof of my mouth.

"My bed is in my house."

"Will you take me to your house sometime?"

"No."

"¿Y porqué no?"

"Because my house is not your business."

I was baffled and felt slighted, but didn't know just why. Wasn't all the servants' business our business? We employed them. We fed them. We clothed them. It was our duty to do it, I'd heard Mami and Daddy say. "Duty," so like "soon," another complicated word. I was silent for a moment, my gaze resting on the curve of nana's back as she leaned into her ironing. Her arm swung back and forth.

"Well, I don't care what you say. One day I'm going to follow you all the way home."

She interrupted the rhythmic cadence of her work and let out one of her puffs. This time it was one that never seemed to end.

About a month later, I tried to do it. The sun was setting, but it was still light as nana headed down the driveway to the bus stop about a block away. She had changed out of her uniform and into her regular clothes. She had put on her shoes, which were like two flat black boats. (At the house, she went barefoot all day.) She carried two large bags filled with heaven knows what. Each day she arrived with these bags; every evening she left with them.

I crept quietly after her, keeping to the fringe of grass that bordered the graveled driveway. I'd shut Chicha up in my bedroom so she wouldn't follow and give me away. There were many people waiting at the bus stop and I tried to lose myself among them. Luckily, the buses came frequently and the wait wasn't long. At this time of day the traffic made a great clatter. Cars whizzed by. Trucks ground their gears; smoke stacks spewed black stinky clouds. I kept an eye on nana and when the bus rolled up and halted in a great hiss of brakes, I followed her up the steps. She was in front of the person in front of me. She slipped into an empty spot at the back of the bus. I pushed my way to her side and surprised her in the aisle. "Nana!"

Her eyes widened and for an instant she was speechless. The bus lurched forward, beginning my long-awaited journey. I was thrilled beyond belief. Nana jumped up. She leaned over the other passengers crowded on the bench. Clutching her bags, she took hold of the thick cord threaded along the top of the bus windows. She gave the string two quick yanks. Not saying a word, she grasped my arm fiercely and elbowed her way through the people crowded in the aisle. The bus came to a halt, and she dragged me down the back steps and onto the ground. When the bus pulled away, she turned me around and whacked me on the rump. I started to cry. "Quiet," she commanded. "I can't believe it. You could be lost." I tried to explain that this could never happen. How could I be lost with her at my side? But nana had no use for explanations. Her hand was a vise around my wrist as she escorted me up the road, down the driveway and into the house.

No one had noticed my disappearance. I slipped into my room and fell onto the bed. Chicha tried to jump up, but her big belly kept her from it. I reached down and hoisted her up. "I wanted to go to nana's house," I lamented. The dream of nana's business, her house, her own bed heaped with the contents of her bags faded into nothingness.

Chicha licked my face. I sucked my thumb.

• • •

In August, because it was fiesta time, school was out for the week and I had the freedom to wander around the property and poke my nose into other people's business. Just like Nancy Drew, I now conducted my own investigations.

I investigated don Tomás and Blanca's house, pretending I was just visiting. Chicha waddled along to keep up. I noted the ramshackle dresser in a corner. The one chair. The bed with boards laid across the frame, but with no mattress on top. The little shelf tacked to the wall. The pictures of saints and the votive candle resting beneath them. In Blanca's cooking shed, I dropped down beside her and watched her make tortillas. If I was lucky, she would pinch off a wad of corn dough and let me turn it against my palm. I tried slapping the dough as she did, but my tortillas were never as round as hers. Still, it was a satisfying thing to set my creation on the hot clay griddle, to watch it puff up and then brown until it was ready. Just like her, I sprinkled my tortilla with salt and then I wolfed it down, pronouncing it la mejor tortilla del mundo, the best tortilla in the world. Blanca beamed when I said this.

That day she was not happy. She squatted at the griddle, her big belly like a basketball resting in her lap. She slapped the dough, her mind obviously elsewhere. At length, I risked a question. "¿Qué le pasa, Blanca? ¿Porque está triste?" Why are you sad?

She gave a shrug, and was silent as if mulling over things. Then she added, "Tomás se fué."

"Where did he go?"

She shrugged again, and though I waited for further explanations, that was the end of it.

Later, when I was in the laundry room sneakily investigating what nana kept in her two big bags, I asked her about don Tomás.

"Who knows where he is," she said, and the answer was most unsatisfactory. "It's just like a man to take off like that." The added bit of information puzzled me, yet it seemed oddly right. Daddy was a man. Daddy had left two days before to go hunting. An idea struck me, like a revelation. "Maybe don Tomás is hunting," I said.

"He's hunting, all right," nana said, and I was proud that my investigative powers had thrown a light on what had been a puzzlement.

A day before Daddy came home from his hunting, don Tomás returned from his. I was at the end of the driveway, investigating the old well behind his house. The well was no longer in use and, over the years, it had filled up with garden clippings and construction debris. I liked to pretend it was an Aztec cenote, a watery reservoir, but instead of imagining water in the hole, I pictured a place where the bodies of sacrificed princesses were laid to rest. I'd been reading a book about the Aztecs and their customs, how a special maiden was chosen for a sacrifice. How her heart was ripped from her chest as an offering. That day, I was poking at the debris with a long stick, hoping to uncover the body of an Aztec maiden with a bloody chest, when I heard don Tomás. Over the wall that circled his house, I could hear him muttering. I flung my stick into the well and raced around the wall to greet him.

Don Tomás sat on a three-legged stool resting beside the door to his house. His head was in his hands. Blanca stood in the doorway, her face set in stone, her arms folded across her big belly.

"Don Tomás!" I exclaimed. "You've come back."

There was joy in my heart. He had left; he'd returned. Daddy, too, would soon return.

Don Tomás lifted his head and gazed at me. His eyes were watery. His cheeks and chin were a rash of stubble. The sight of him, so wretched, took me aback. His shirt and trousers were a mess. He was wearing only one shoe. He smelled like a cotton ball when Mami placed it against the rubbing-alcohol bottle.

"Don Tomás, ¿qué le paso?"

He shook his head. Blanca said nothing.

I squatted down beside him. Looked up into his rheumy eyes. "What happened, don Tomás?"

After some consideration, he said, "Me caí de un palo'e coco." I fell out of a coconut tree.

I jumped up in alarm. "Uy, pobrecito!" You poor thing. I pictured him tumbling down from a great height to the ground, coconuts crashing down after, maybe one bonking him on the head. "I'll go get my mother," I said. Mami had a first aid kit she kept in the closet, next to the strongbox, next to the guns.

Don Tomás sprung up from the stool, reaching immediately to steady himself against the wall. "No, no, no. Ya voy a'star bien." I'll be all right.

Blanca came to me and took my hand. She said, "Come, don't worry about him. I'll walk you home."

We trudged down the driveway, toward the house. We said nothing on the way. Somehow, I knew to say nothing when I arrived.

• • •

Soon after, my parents threw a party. All the lights in the house were on, and the place looked like a lit birthday cake. Three guitarists stood together and strummed popular tunes. My sister Ani and I had been allowed to stay up and greet the guests. Most were embassy people, and they crowded the living room and the porch. The men wore dark suits; the women were glamorous in their long dresses, their shoulders bared, jewels circling their necks and dangling from their ears. All held cocktail glasses and as the contents went down, spirits rose up.

The dining table and buffet were laid with platters filled with tamalitos de sal, pupusas, curtido, yuca frita, and quesos frescos, all awaiting the main fare for the night: the wild pig swabbed with oil and aromatic herbs and roasting slowly above the bed of red-hot coals out in the yard. Don Tomás was tending to the roast. Earlier in the day, he'd dug the pit for the fire and constructed the spit to hold the pig. Blanca and Juana were dressed in crisp white uniforms; they wove their way among the guests with trays of drinks and canapés.

I was sitting on the steps that led down from the porch, observing what transpired. I watched Mami and how captivating she looked in her midnight blue dress with the scalloped hem. She went from guest to guest, a drink in her hand, her face radiant. I watched Daddy tell a cluster of men about how he shot the pig. The pig in question was a pitiful sight and it made me sad. It was stretched out along the spit as if it were still running. It turned over and over again. I watched don Tomás swab the pig with the new cotton mop purchased just for the occasion. Don Tomás's face was lit by the embers and his face glowed like a scary mask. I watched the Marine, one of the embassy sentinels, who sat on the low-wall of the porch. He was in his blue uniform and had a crew cut. I watched a large woman wearing a long tight dress that made her look like a fat sausage. She clapped her hands to the beat of guitars. She stamped her feet like a flamenco dancer. Encouraged by the crowd's approval, she placed a filled cocktail glass on her head and balanced it there as she pranced around. I watched in fascination, thinking that at any moment the glass would teeter and Johnny Walker whiskey would cascade down her head, but this did not occur.

Disappointed, I left the porch and went through the kitchen and out into the laundry room. The party clatter was subdued there and the light was low. I went over to the corner, by the water heater, to the big cardboard box lined with paper excelsior and with the opening carved out of the side. Chicha looked up at me in greeting. Her six little pups were nestled against her. When I picked up one of her babies and cuddled it, she thumped her tail against the side of the box. The pup was a tiny bundle of warmth. I gave it little kisses, and it opened its mouth in delight, its breath moist and heavenly.

• • •

On March 21, 1951, five days before my tenth birthday, Daddy received Form FS-349, his transfer papers. Mexico City would be our next post. His new ambassador would be the Honorable William O'Dwyer, formerly His Honor, Mayor of New York City. Daddy wrote the obligatory letter: "My dear Mr. Ambassador, I am pleased to report that I am preparing to leave this post and expect to arrive in Mexico about April 8th . . . "

We had been evicted from our countryside paradise. We were bereft. I thought of Nancy Drew and how she might answer this question that had so cruelly interfered with our tranquility: When life is serene and rich and joyful, why does paradise not last forever?

• • •

In Mexico, we started a new life. A few years later, this life began to feel like another kind of paradise. But unlike the one we'd made at La Ceiba, our Mexican paradise was colorful, wild and dramatic, mostly on account of our second cousins.

Olivia, Emilia and Marisol were the daughters of my mother's cousin, tía Clara. The two younger girls were my and Ani's ages. The family was large and extended and they all had squeezed into a stone house built by their father, Federico Fuentes, in one of Mexico City's quiet neighborhoods. Federico Fuentes was a frustrated actor who had a zeal for wearing costumes to parties and sometimes, if it suited his purposes, to business meetings. He'd once showed up for one in full field marshal's regalia: the braid, the epaulettes, the stars. He was presently engaged in building houses, and the convolutions of what he did were swathed in intrigue, something not atypical when it comes to doing business in los Estados Unidos de Mexico.

Federico Fuentes's success had everything to do with his suave demeanor and his grand persuasive skills. Splendid in a uniform, his blue-black hair slicked back under a be-ribboned military cap, Federico Fuentes could talk a dead man into rising. True to his nature, when Federico began constructing houses, he deftly acquired his building materials by militarily "requisitioning" them from the Mexican Government. Adding best fortune to good, he enjoined personnel from the Army to serve as construction workers; all this labor, of course, not chargeable to him. It was simply unbelievable and utterly Mexican. And so houses went up, communities bloomed and multiplied and everyone was happy. Most specially Federico

Fuentes who, contrary to the axiom "it takes money to make money," could make money from ingenuity alone.

My cousins' living room looked out upon a narrow front yard separated from the street by a concrete wall crowned with shards of broken glass (to keep thieves from climbing over) and a wide iron gate at the driveway. At thirteen, Olivia was the oldest of the cousins, and she had a novio, a boyfriend, who, when he came around, gave a little whistle. When she heard him, Olivia would throw up her hands and visibly tremble. Usually, her sister Emilia had to catch her before her knees buckled, but Ani and I would hotfoot it to the living room, skootching sideways around the huge architectural maquette that Federico Fuentes had placed upon the dining table a year back, a maquette that stretched from wall to wall, totally negating the functionality of the living and dining rooms. My sister and I knelt on the sofa and craned our necks, the better to see out the window and over the wall; the better to catch a glimpse of the top of el novio's head. From our high vantage point, it appeared that he had slicked-back hair, just like Federico Fuentes.

We'd watch Olivia stride out to the gate, her belled-out skirt sashaying as she went. We'd watch her come to the gate, a black iron bastion her father had had built with his daughters in mind. The gate kept them in the compound, away from worldliness and thus, from temptation. Still, from the window, Ani and I could hear the love words el novio propelled like blazing arrows over Federico Fuentes's rampart. "Mi cielo. Mi corazón. Mi encanto. Mi vida." My heaven. My heart. My enchantment. My life.

Oh, the red-hot vividness of love words voiced in Spanish.

• • •

Intrepidly à la mode, and because no meals could be taken in the dining room, Federico Fuentes had built a booth in the kitchen, a replica of drug store Americana, all red vinyl and chrome. He'd become enamored of just such a booth when he and tía Clara lived in Nueva York and he was acting on "Broway." If you asked enough times, you'd eventually learn that this was not the Great White Way, but some place in the Bronx no map seemed to include.

Federico Fuentes's kitchen booth was a visual surprise, and each banquette was inches shy of the combined width of the fannies attempting to sit there. Before meals everyone tried not to be the one who had to scoot over to be pressed against the wall. Olivia never had to do it. "I might need to use the bathroom," she'd say, mysteriously evasive. Because she had recently become what tía Clara called, "una mujer," a woman, Olivia always got her way. Being the youngest of the bunch, it was usually my sister and Marisol who had to take the wall positions.

One day, as always, the women of the house were having lunch before the master of the house arrived for his. We were packed in the booth, the cook setting before us on the gray-speckled tabletop bowls of asopao, a hearty rice soup. Because of our proximity, the air was rife with the bitter odor of asafetida. The foul-smelling roots were packed into little cloth bags and hung with string around each of our necks. It was 1953 and everywhere there was the threat of poliomyelitis. We were to wear our little bags, no matter how much they reeked, as protection against the disease. We were not to use the public swimming pools, nor heaven forbid, the public rest rooms. We were not to linger in crowds. All needless prohibitions given the presence of that great iron gate.

I plunged a spoon into my soup, my eyes and ears open to new tensions vibrating around us. Federico Fuentes's mother had come and gone after a substantial visit. I never had the occasion to meet her, being that my sister and I always arrived just after the mother-in-law had left, or we left just before she arrived. But we hadn't missed the house histrionics that preceded or followed her visits.

Tía Clara blasphemed, her dark eyes blazing. "She's a witch, a witch!" Tía Clara's mother, tía Julia (my own grandmother's sister), hurried around the house with her ubiquitous bottle of holy water, liberally sprinkling every nook and cranny to wash away her daughter's imprecations, the threat of polio and any lingering witch aura.

At the moment, tía Julia, a small bent-back woman who wore nothing but black, was in the kitchen, at the booth, dousing us all as we tried to eat. She rolled her eyes upward in silent imploration as she shook water over us.

"Aquí, Mámi, aquí," tía Clara urged, reaching out with her right hand, the actual hand that had touched the witch. Tía Julia poured a puddle into her palm and then massaged her daughter's hand and all five fingers, not stopping at that, but continuing past her wrist (the one with all the silver bracelets) and up her arm, the exorcism ending at the crook of the elbow. "¡Ay, Hija, ay!" tía Julia murmured, her eyes rolling up and up as if it were the devil himself who had stepped into the house to leave behind his evilness.

"What did she do?" I asked, because, like Nancy Drew, I was very interested in particulars.

"What did who do?" Berta, tía Clara's sister, retorted, talking around the ever-present cigarette in her mouth. Tía Berta was a tall spinster who, like her mother, was enamored of wearing black. Unlike tía Clara, who wore her hair in a froth around her face, tía Berta's hair was pulled severely back into a bun. With her left hand, she withdrew the cigarette from her mouth for only the moment it took to have three spoonfuls of soup.

"¿La bruja?" I said. "What did the witch do?" I couldn't help recalling the story of la Ziguanaba, nana's old story. That wailing woman had always seemed like a witch to me.

Tía Clara pinned me with a glare. "What *didn't* she do, that's the question!"

I turned back to my soup. I was twelve, and I understood that there were limits to a girl's inquisitiveness. The subject was closed; the place had been cleansed; the dust of familial discontent had been dampened.

But in my mind spun a whirlwind of possibilities. The "what ifs," the "how comes," the "why nots." I often posed these questions to myself no matter what the situation. I didn't know it back then, but I was learning to be a writer.

• • •

At the end of the cousins' driveway (a place we used for endless rounds of roller skating) stood the theater that Federico Fuentes had fashioned from the garage, and which he named after his youngest daughter. "Cine Marisol" was emblazoned on a marquee above the door.

The theater had a projection booth, a dressing and makeup room with a huge mirror, a wide silver screen that pulled down over an actual proscenium stage. Four rows of seats fronted the stage, twenty seats in all, each requisitioned from the Mexican movie industry.

Recently, I'd had a personal revelation: I was convinced that I was a famous movie star, that my life was being played out on a screen as I lived it, that when I died the curtain would drop and the audience would stand and deliver an ovation. This belief was bolstered by my family's personal acquaintance with two famous Mexican movie stars: my sister's godparents were the legendary Fernando and Mapy Cortez.

El Cine Marisol itself had me dreaming about fame. I liked to stand on the stage and give rousing performances. To prepare myself, I'd sit on the tall chair in the dressing room and gaze into the mirror lighted by little white bulbs. Sometimes I stared at myself so intently that my vision blurred and it was then that I pretended to be my twin sister, Susana. I pretended that it had been me who had expired in Washington, D.C. When I lost myself like this, I sometimes spent the whole day pretending to be who I was not. But this secret I kept to myself lest tía Julia come after me with the holy water.

I always started my performances with a magical phrase, slowly raising my arms and dramatically declaring: "Se levanta el telón." The curtain goes up. No curtain graced el Cine Marisol stage, Federico Fuentes's only oversight, hence the need for such visual clarification. While on stage this day, my sister was my only audience. Though Ani was ten and a half, she still obeyed my every command.

Not too long before, we had both clambered up to the roof of the small shed tucked into the back corner of our house's yard. I handed her an umbrella and ordered her to open it and jump to the ground. I had read about such a feat in a book and thought it would be a fine experience to see the feat performed. "No. Por favor, no," Ani whimpered, clutching the opened umbrella as if it were a lifeline. But I set my face and fixed her with a look as fierce as tía Clara's and Ani had no choice but to leap into space. Luckily for us both, the distance to the ground was not great and other than being shaken, she landed without harm.

I was not aware of this then, but when I set my mind to it, I can be an ugly girl.

In any case, that day, Ani had been sweeping back and forth in her roller skates over the cousins' driveway while I was in the dressing room staring hard into the mirror and becoming Susana. When the transformation was complete, I requisitioned Ani for my audience. She sat there now, her skates still clamped to her shoes, her hands bunched in her lap, her startling blue eyes turned up to me.

"Se levanta el telón," I started, speaking in Spanish as I always did, then adding my second opening phrase: "Había una vez."

"Once upon a time, there was a lady who looked like a witch. She had stringy hair down to her waist and long pointy fingernails that could dig into you. The witch was very mean, mala mala mean, and she had a baby she didn't want, so she threw it away. Now the witch is sorry, and she screams and yells and pulls out her hair . . . "

On stage at el Cine Marisol and because I was now

Susana, I let loose like a banshee. It was liberating to do it. But to do it, I had to become someone else.

• • •

A year later, Daddy became disenchanted with the Foreign Service, where he saw no happy future for himself, so he resigned. We would move back to El Salvador where he would go into the flower-growing business. As agricultural attaché, Daddy had visited various gladiola plantations to investigate and report on the production and export of cut flowers to the United States. This aspect of horticulture had begun to make a significant impression in U.S. import figures. The success of gladiola cultivation in particular had Daddy asking himself, Why not join in the parade? So it was decided. Sadly, but without complaints, Mami closed up the house in Mexico City. She put behind her the affable society that was embassy life: the teas, the cocktail receptions and her beloved bridge-playing get-togethers. To fund the new adventure, she and Daddy cashed in their assets, including all the furniture. Ani and I were once again pulled out of school. Until the business was going, Mami, my sister and I would move in with Mami's parents in Santurce, Puerto Rico. We'd be enrolled in a new school. Filled with anticipation, Daddy went off to El Salvador to launch our new life. When the time was right, he would send for us.

Abuelito and Abuelita joyfully took us in. Though our separation from Daddy had been a teary one, reunion with family was a balm for unhappiness. The shift from a burgeoning and bustling metropolis to the provincial, unhurried way of Puerto Rican life was a welcomed change. Abuelito Celestino exemplified island living. He was a slender, shy man, a man of little words who awakened slowly with little to say and who retired with even less to add. Every morning, after a leisurely breakfast, he strolled to his law office, a few blocks away. In contrast, Abuelita Marina was a whirlwind around Abuelito's placidity. She was a stout woman with a regal bearing and plenty of opinions. As she scurried about, nothing escaped her eye or ear. Her domain was a six-room apartment on the building's third floor. In addition, there was an open-to-the-elements veranda and a balcony from which you could keep an eye on the street and the neighbors' goings-on.

In Abuelita's realm there was a world of chores: the servants had to be managed and directed, the laundry readied, the meals planned, the shopping detailed in lengthy lists. Abuelita's sewing basket, a woven container plump and round as a large melon, sat beside her easy chair awaiting her busy hands. Even in the easy chair, she was never at rest. She read in the chair. Sewed in the chair. Gave commands from the chair. Mami was equally industrious. Almost immediately upon arriving, she'd found employment as a secretary for a shipping company in San Juan. Every weekday morning, she walked to the corner with Abuelito and then parted company with him when she climbed aboard the bus.

The apartment was spacious enough to comfortably house the five of us. Ani and I shared a bedroom and Mami had one of her own. Over all the beds, mosquito nets cascaded from hoops set into the ceiling. During the day, each net was wound into a single plait and gathered up into a loose knot. At night, each was undone and tucked tightly around its mattress.

Lying in bed, waiting for sleep (a girl can sleep better when her father's in the house), the world appeared milky in a maze of gauze. Still, I knew the room by heart: the dainty desk with legs as slender as a colt's, the floor lamp with its fringed shade, the tall five-drawer dresser with the rosette pulls. And hanging on the wall in the space between the beds, the gilt-framed image of a great-winged angel hovering above two children crossing a roaring river over a rickety bridge.

Oftentimes, I felt as if I too stood on a perilous bridge, my ears filled with the ominous sound of rushing water. At night, in Puerto Rico, my heart ached for that graveled driveway under the coconut palms, for that old foundation housing my imaginary castle, for that broad flat rock where I sat to soak in the sun. For nana, too, whose very flesh was imbued with the scent of pressed cotton. For the servants' oak table, overspread with tender stories. Behind the gauzy veil surrounding my bed, that paradise had all but vanished. When these thoughts struck and kept sleep away, I'd slip my thumb into my mouth and picture a wide-winged angel named Susana watching over me.

• • •

At the abuelitos' house, I did my homework after school on the veranda. I often eschewed the desk that was there, preferring to sit on the daybed covered prettily in flowered chintz and with pillows plumped against the wall. Though the day might be hot, the ceiling fan created a breeze. One day, I was working on the last of a natural science project: we were to select either fauna or flora, write a paper, fill a notebook with illustrations. For my project, I'd chosen el colibrí, the hummingbird, because it was the island's most beloved bird and because Abuelito had a magazine featuring them and he'd given me permission to use the pictures for cutouts. To do it, Abuelita allowed me to use her little curved scissors. I selected a number of bird varieties: the band-tailed barbthroat, the white-bellied emerald, the purple-crown fairy, the white-tailed, the violet-eared, the green-breasted hummingbird. Against the far wall of the veranda, a trellis exuberantly spilled flowering jasmine and the colibrís came frequently to drink in the fragrant nectar. I watched them hover, dart backward, forward and sideways. The blur of wings enchanted me. They appeared so joyful, catching sweetness where they could.

Perched on the daybed, I carefully snipped away while keeping an ear to what was coming over the radio that set on a nearby table. That afternoon, there was more news about "el moreno de Bayamon," the convict who'd escaped as he was being transported to jail. For days, the newspaper had carried stories about the man's murderous rampage. It seemed he had used a carving knife to butcher three people. The paper had carried the victims' photos. In one of them—luckily, it was black and white—you could see lots of blood. A fourth victim was in the hospital, but not expected to live. It was this man who croaked, "fué el moreno de Bayamon," it was the black man from Bayamon, before they wheeled him into surgery. On the radio, music programs, and even soap operas, were interrupted with updates of sightings. El moreno was in Guaynabo. In Caguas. In Carolina.

It was my belief that if the man could be in all those places, he could also be in Santurce. So near, in fact, he might, at any time, throw a leg over the balcony (no matter that our apartment was three-floors up) and slash me to confetti with his big knife.

I'd voiced my fear to Abuelita because being cut was my worst fear, but she informed me I was being silly. She said the man was wearing handcuffs when he escaped and was incapable of anything. I was not too sure, but the news eased my concern. I said nothing to Mami, for she had to ride the bus to and from work, and I didn't want to alarm her with fears that el moreno might somehow be able to commandeer her bus, single her out and hack her to pieces. This thought had kept me tossing at night. When I told my sister, she rolled her blue eyes and said, "Ay, mi hermana 'sta loca." I said nothing, because I was not crazy, though I could see how it was entirely possible for a person to go crazy with a brain swirling with carving knives.

That day, Mami strolled onto the veranda, having arrived from work. She wore a mint-green linen dress and spectator pumps. She smelled as sweet as jasmine. I was so relieved to see her, I jumped up and spilled my homework. "What's this," she asked, retrieving a few of the cutouts I was readying to paste up.

"Colibrís, Mami. They're for my science project. It's due tomorrow."

"Que lindos." She handed the pretty things over, then leaned over the balcony and called out "Yohoo!" Soon an echoing "Yohoo!" came from below. It was Toñin, who lived beneath us and who was Mami's best friend. "I'll be right down," Mami called to her.

I was disappointed for I was hoping to have my mother's company. Had hoped she might even help me with my cutouts. I had six to go. Mami gave me a quick kiss and went off to see her friend. I dragged a chair over to the balcony because I knew the two would be soon chatting directly under me and I might catch snatches of their conversation. That day, I wished I hadn't been such a snoop. Mami told Toñin there had been news from Daddy. His flower business was not doing very well. In fact, Mami said, he might have to shut it down. "What then?" Toñin had asked. "I don't know," Mami replied.

The news had shaken me so, I abandoned my homework, not caring that, when morning came, my project would be unfinished. I escaped to my room, my bed, unfastening the mosquito net so that it fell around me. I needed the comfort of a vaporous world, for the implications of what was happening to my father I could not understand. Besides, I could feel disaster lurking as surely as if el moreno himself were stealthily making his way up the back steps of our apartment.

In the morning, after Mami had left for work and I slumped out to the breakfast table, my notebook rested beside my plate. I opened it and found that all my missing hummingbirds had been pasted in. Under each was a caption of the bird's name in Spanish and in Latin. Also included were each bird's field mark, voice and range. A little note from Mami was clipped at the top: Darling, you looked so tired last night that I thought I'd lend you a hand. Kisses, Mami.

• • •

Not long after, the radio blared that el moreno was back in Bayamon, his home town, and was trapped in a cornfield as vast as an airfield. The police had circled the field and shouted directives over bullhorns. "We have you surrounded! Come out of there at once!"

A crop-duster flew over and let loose a cloud of insecticide. The plane made a number of passes. El moreno held his ground. It seemed like all the island was tuned to the drama unfolding over the radio. We were no different. The radio on the veranda brought us updates, interviews of relatives, including his mother, who tearfully urged her son to give up. "Dáte por vencido, mi hijo. Te lo suplico por favor." Give up, my son. I beg of you, please. Her imploration was taped and the police blared it again and again over the cornfield. I listened, both mesmerized and terrified. I pictured a man choking back white dust. A man in handcuffs with arms caught behind his back. A man eaten alive by insects. A man rubbed raw by the sharpness of corn stalks. Still, he had committed a horrible crime. Three people had died under his knife, and there was the fourth now, for the man in the hospital had finally succumbed.

The day after, the police acted in a way that stunned me. They set fire to the perimeter of the cornfield, hoping to roust el moreno out. Within minutes, the conflagration was so swift that the radio announcer declared you could see the fire out to sea. Over the radio there came a sound like a wind rushing out of control. Over the radio, came crackling and popping.

Since that day in Puerto Rico when I was merely twelve, the whole of that incident left a deep impression. In the end, I couldn't reconcile what el moreno had done with what had been done to him. Ultimately, it was the puzzling out of this type of conundrum that would form the heart of what I came to write.

• • •

With such riddles filling my head, was it any wonder then, that my tummy problems started up again? Following the logic that, where the alimentary canal is concerned, what goes in, must eventually come out, I became a picky eater. It made sense that the less I ate, the shorter my bathroom stays. Of course, this stance of mine had its consequences. Abuelita was forever enticing me to eat, "Coma, Sandy, coma." But I only picked at my food and consequently grew thin, though not dangerously so. Eventually, I came down with anemia and turned pale and lethargic. Concerned, Mami took me to the doctor on her day off from work, and after an examination of my nail beds and the inside of my lower eyelids, he prescribed a series of iron shots. The doctor arranged for a pharmacist (on the island, all pharmacists gave injections) to come to the apartment once a week for my treatments.

El señor Romero came on Tuesdays, at three. When I arrived from school, I fell into Abuelita's arms and started to bawl. My sister changed out of her school uniform and made herself scarce, but I, whimpering and cajoling all the while, trailed Abuelita as she lighted the votive candle to the Arcángel San Rafael, her favorite saint and the patron of druggists and of healing, as she heated up a towel in the oven to use as a compress for the pain I'd soon endure, for indeed, iron shots are painful. The medication to be delivered is thick and dark as chocolate syrup and must be injected deeply into the muscle, slowly, to be sure it is absorbed.

Each Tuesday, my grandparents' wide bed provided the torture site. I'd dodge the druggist, until he corralled me into the bedroom; I'd holler for mercy, while el señor, holding aloft his gigantic syringe, exhorted Abuelita to pull my panties down and lay me on the bed, across her lap. Thus positioned, my bare buttocks splotched dark from the druggist's previous assaults, he would set upon them again. As always, I gathered fistfuls of bedspread and held on for dear life. As always, I wailed like la Ziguanaba, my tears so copious they slid down my cheeks and fell upon the bedspread's blue shantung, turning it the hue of stormy skies.

Abuelita, one hand over my thighs, the other spread over my back to keep me still, matched my laments.

"¡Ay, Abuelita, ay!" I bellowed.

"¡Ay, hija, ay!" she echoed.

In unison, we cried. Me for my misery, she for it as well.

I ask you, in all this world, is there a purer form of consolation?

• • •

Eight months later, my father sent for us and we left Puerto Rico and moved back to San Salvador and into a number of houses and neighborhoods, none of them possessing the idyllic charm of our little paradise at La Ceiba. Eventually, we settled into a nice two-storied house set on a corner lot of Avenida Olímpica, just blocks away from El Salvador del Mundo, the hub of our city district: a grassy public square that featured at its center the statue of Our Saviour standing atop the world, His arms open wide in blessing.

Not defeated by the failure of his gladiola business, Daddy eventually started up an earth-moving company, which fortunately prospered and allowed him to be somewhat of a Missouri farm-boy again as he worked with his massive tractors and loaders and graters. For his company car, he purchased an orange VW and had his logo painted on each front door: a circle the bright color of his Beetle, with "Jimmy Ables y Cia." printed over the image of a Caterpillar D-9, its huge tires, transformed into earth-uprooting paws, its wide grill converted into a fierce toothy grin that shouted, "There is nothing I can't do."

Before he and Mami moved back to the States in 1962, Jimmy Ables and Company owned a fleet of those orange Beatles.

For all his years, the same ferocious tenacity pictured on his logo fueled my father's life. He was never ruled by money nor cowed by the lack of it; for that, there was my mother and thus her periodic anxiety as she opened the strongbox stashed in the closet beside her shoes. Being the adventuresome man he was, my father was ever curious and willing to turn the corner of whatever safe haven of a street he happened to be living on to take off into the unknown and the headwind of uncertainty. As ever, Mami trailed behind him. Before he died he confessed to me that, in his life, his only deep preoccupation had been my mother's preoccupations. Still, though he was ever her faithful and true companion, he'd been either unwilling or not able to give her the only thing she truly craved: a permanent home, a place to set down roots that would spread, tough and strong, under her. Roots to keep her from toppling over.

In the almost sixty years that they were married, my parents had lived in close to thirty homes.

• • •

In the surgery room at Abbott Northwestern Hospital, Dr. Madoff perhaps has just made the incision over nurse Susie's X-marks-the-spot. Perhaps he has begun to lift the slippery end of my small intestine up through the opening and will soon be turning the intestine over like a cuffed-sock before stitching it to my belly. I, thank the Lord, am oblivious to this. In the white haze of anesthesia, I'll soon be leaving El Salvador and heading off to Missouri.

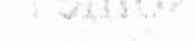

IN 1955, WHEN I WAS FOURTEEN, Daddy sent me abroad to attend high school. He was hoping, he said, to "Americanize" me and, as a bonus, I'm sure, to break me of the habit of being served. The prospect of such a journey thrilled me, implying a future filled with adventure. But at the same time, I grew melancholy at the thought of leaving. Late at night, I'd gaze out the window that was set just above my bed. Out there, up the avenida, glowed the lighted statue of el Salvador del Mundo. I'd think, What will become of me so far away from home? In my father's defense, this sending-away was not unusual. Most of my schoolmates were also off to the United States, some to Europe, for education and refinement in boarding and finishing schools, much like the English, who have been sending their children away for centuries.

No boarding school for me. I was sent to Missouri, to live with Grandma Hazel, Daddy's mother, and Grandpa Orion, his stepfather, on their small dairy farm.

No servants there. The farm stood on the outskirts of Unionville, a town in the northeastern part of the state with a population of less than 2,000. At my father's request, my grandma and grandpa gladly and graciously took me in. They lived in the ancestral home built before the Civil War, a house that sat back where the old road had once been, back past the barn and the implement shed and the corncrib. But this was in the mid-fifties, a time of new prosperity, and when I arrived, the family was in the process of planning the new house, which they would industriously build themselves. A house by the side of the new county road. A house that would possess all the conveniences the present house did not: an automatic furnace in a real basement, running water from taps, an indoor bathroom with a tub, a gas oven and stove. A dream house for certain, but a dream that was at least a year away from coming true.

Over the fifty years that have passed since I was fourteen, I've often marveled at how agreeable I'd been to allow myself to be banished from the lap of luxury to the hardscrabble life of the farm. While my mother's ailments intensified after my father's pronouncement, I went blithely off to the land of Archie and Veronica, to the land of dungarees and cardigans, to the land of penny loafers worn with white-cuffed ankle socks.

And while I finally did discover these things and found them to be entrancing, it's also true that I found something quite different as well.

I found the old house. Prim as a spinster, it sat atop a hill, stoic and resigned. Narrow and two-storied, its outer walls were rough to the touch and the color of pigeon wings. Inside, a claw-foot dining table and spindle-back chairs lent grace to the front room; beyond it lay grandma and grandpa's bedroom with the pretty curtains serving for doors. The living room contained what amounted to two wonders of the world to an El Salvador-reared girl: the hulking wood-burning stove with its shiny nickel-capped corners and its isinglass door, and best of all, the Sylvania television set, a rarity in Central America.

The bosom of the house was the kitchen, of course, and it featured a big cast-iron cook-stove with round cook-plates under which fires were kept lit from dawn to late into the night. At one side was the reservoir, a deep well that held the house's only constant supply of hot water. In fact, the house had no running water at all. For that, water was lugged in by arm-numbing buckets from the pump out by the barn. In addition, set against a wall, and next to the door that opened onto the utility porch, was another of the room's grand contraptions, the cream separator with its gleaming metal exterior, its large pans, one atop the other, the puzzling maze of tubes joining the two. Next to the family's herd of Guernseys, the separator was the heart of their dairy farm's operation.

Set in an alcove of the kitchen was the family's wash station: towel and washcloth draped over a rack, a wide ledge that held a large pitcher, that you could fill up at the reservoir, and a deep bowl, plus the dish cradling the Naptha bar. The more fastidious and personal washing I'd accomplished by taking the bowl and soap to my room.

I slept upstairs, in a long room with low slanting walls that conformed to the pitch of the roof. A room far away from the downstairs heat source. To keep me from freezing, grandma would spread my bed with her homemade down comforter, a true luxury. Each night, she readied two rubber bottles, both filled with hot water from the stove's reservoir. One to place at my feet, the other to snuggle with. Great comforts, much like nana's warm ironing-cloth on my tummy, like abuelita's wailing as I took those torturous iron shots. At grandma's house those winter nights, I'd burrow into her comforter, curl my toes around the hot water bottle and listen to the moan of the wind, to the way it sometimes set the plastic stretched across the windows to whistling. I'd picture the snow banked against the house and out along the fences grandpa seemed always to be mending. I'd picture the cattle huddled together in the barn. I'd imagine the ewes in the sheep shed and strained to hear their woeful bleating. Some nights, it was the cry of la Ziguanaba that I heard instead.

• • •

Despite the novelty of my surroundings, despite the spate of new adventures, the bathroom situation, the lack thereof, was a matter of concern. Given my propensity for bathroom occupation, this kind of adventure did not sit too well with me. Consider this: during the day and in good weather, I had to use the ever-redolent outhouse, with the only light coming through the half-moon grandpa'd carved at the top of the door. The outhouse with its two frightening openings: one to sit over, the other yawning beside me. Both caused me worry, sometimes even terror. I'd sit gingerly down, thinking, something's down there in that stinky darkness! Something from down there's going to crawl up my butt! Needless to say, there was never any tarrying in the outhouse for me. Actually, I learned to "hold it," waiting to use the school facilities, or the bathrooms at friends' houses. It goes without saying, that this habit does not do wonders for the gut.

In addition, during bad weather (storms, tornado threats, snow, ice), when getting to the outhouse was impossible, and during the night when it was too dark to make my way, there was the "thunder" bucket, a white porcelain pot with a wide lip for sitting and a lid to fit over. This was stashed under my bed.

All in all, the comparison of what I'd left behind and what I had come to was nothing short of staggering. I think about the description in that old medical symptoms book, and while it's now understood that UC and other IBDs, such as Crohn's disease, are not a result of personality quirks—but are perhaps linked to the immune system and antibodies gone amok—there might have been something to the belief that emotional upsets could contribute to the problem. Looking back, perhaps there had been a weak spot in my gut after all. I know for sure that there was one in my heart. Try as I might to hide it from myself, my heart was a wee bit broken. Was I not separated from my parents and my sister (I would never live full-time with them again), from my friends, from nana, from Chicha, our family dog? Was I not now far away from all my familiar and comforting possessions: my bed, my tub, my toilet bowl? From El Salvador itself, a country I'd grown to love as my own?

To compound my loss, communication from home was infrequent, given the unreliability of the Salvadoran postal service, given that the cost of telephone calls from Central America to Missouri was exorbitant.

As was my way, I never spoke of these things, never

discussed them with grandma. But she was astute and nosed them out. Her sympathy I observed in what she did for me, in the chores she did not burden me with. As she did for the rest of the family, grandma cooked and ironed and washed for me. Because we had no running water, the wash was especially burdensome: water hauled in buckets from the pump, water heated on the stove, clothing run through the hand wringer, and no matter the weather, clothing hung out in the yard. Grandma never asked for my help when she performed these chores, and I, spoiled as I ever was, never volunteered. Clean, freshly ironed clothes set out upon my bed was an expectation. On the farm, as well as back at home.

My measly contributions to the workload were to sometimes dry the supper dishes; when the mood struck, and because I found it entertaining, I'd take a pan and go out to the hen house and collect the eggs. Or I might go out to the field and holler for the cows, maybe even amble out to the animal yard and slop the hogs. Grandma never once complained about my lackadaisical ways. She spoiled me further by allowing me to keep to my bed when the rest of the house was up and out in the barn by five. She did not suggest I help milk the cows, or lend a hand each morning with the tedious work of keeping the separator clean, an important job when it's raw milk being handled.

But there was one thing grandma did insist I do. If I used my thunder bucket, it was my job to empty it. From start to finish, caring for the bucket was an art form, and it took me a few tries to get the process right. First, you add a bit of water to the empty pot, same as there is in our own toilet bowls. Use your imagination and you'll know it's a must. Second, when emptying the pot—in our case, way out across the yard, and over into the ravine that the old road had become—you might want to check the direction of the wind.

One morning, dressed and ready for school, I spotted the school bus off across the ridge. I ran out to the ravine and flung fast and wide. Seconds later, I was wearing the contents of my pot.

I still vividly remember that bright April morning, that eye-widening backsplash. An early metaphor, perhaps, of what I'd be dealing with in the years to come.

• • •

Back in El Salvador, Daddy was busy building roads and dams, terraces and a golf course. Business was so good, in fact, that when I was seventeen and home for the summer, my sister Ani and I were able to make our debut. It was a splendid affair at the country club, both of us dressed in long white gowns as if we were brides. There is a photo of me taken that night, a photo I keep on my dresser. I am in a strapless peau de soie gown standing sideways before a mirror, which casts a double image. Ah, two Sandys, you might think. One the mirror image of the other. But I know the truth. It's not two Sandys. That's me there with Susana.

My escort that night was Jay, who, like me, studied in the States and came home to his family for the summers. He was a few years older than I, and enrolled at USC. We became close after the debut ball and a few weeks after, we were at my house. I was very grown up, I thought, and to prove it, I was throwing a Saturday afternoon party. Our group was enjoying Scotch and waters out by the small pool in the patio, off the living room. My parents were away enjoying, no doubt, their own party at a friend's house, testing their own capacity for Johnny Walkers.

The evening before, Jay and I had been to an American embassy reception for the Yale "Eli Choir." We had stood listening while the handsome young men were stacked along a staircase, serenading the guests with the "Whiffenpoof" song and "Across the Wide Missouri." The embassy butlers wove through the crowd with silver trays laden with cocktails: Scotches, of course, but also martinis and Manhattans. I had lifted a martini from the tray because Jay had chosen one. Also, because the delicate fluted glass charmed me.

That first sip had taken my breath away. My tongue and throat were on fire. Only decorum kept me from spitting the liquid out. Watching my eyes bulge, Jay asked if I was okay. Before he could attempt a pat on my back, I'd brought a gloved hand to my lips. "Of course, I'm okay," I'd sputtered.

Out by the pool, I was very much okay. The two Scotches (no martini-makings at our house) I'd had had numbed my lips and elevated my mood. As the grownups liked to say, I was feeling no pain. We had cranked up the stereo in the living room. La Sonora Matancera, one of the popular bands, was playing a hot merengue. Out on the patio, we all wiggled our hips, lifted our arms to the loud rhythms coming from inside. The afternoon was steamy, but we danced with vigor, stoked by our Scotches, the music, each other.

I was wearing a white piqué sheath our seamstress had finished the day before. Under it, my lacy corselet had narrowed my waist into an hourglass. I could feel the sweat slipping down my back, could feel it pooling in the little hollow between my breasts. I had kicked off my heels and was shredding the bottom of my nylons as I danced on the flagstone. Whatever I was doing to the soles of my feet, did not concern me. I was my own drum; the beat of the music reverberating inside me. My mind was soft and dreamy. I was young. I was a beautiful creature cavorting against a backdrop of mauve bougainvillea frothing down a patio wall. Far away was the reality of the farm, the barn, the sheds, the two-seater outhouse. On the other side of my world was grandma's sturdy kitchen table with its oilcloth draped over, the one printed with square salt and pepper shakers made of green glass. Far away was grandma's Hoosier cabinet with its deep flour bin and the wire racks holding shakers of cinnamon, nutmeg and clove. With its shelves upon which sat the stacks of ironstone dinnerware.

That summer day in El Salvador, my friends and I were dancing out by the pool, when one of the servants materialized from the living room. She motioned me over and I floated over to her.

"There's someone at the door," she said.

"Who?"

She would not say who, only, "He won't come in. He says he wants to talk to you."

I padded off across the red tiles of the living room and then the foyer. I opened the front door to an old friend. "What are you doing here," I asked, perturbed that he was interrupting my idyllic afternoon.

"I've come to stop the music," he said. He lived nearby. There was no car at the curb, so perhaps he'd walked over.

"You can't do that," I told him. Thinking back on this, it is possible I stomped my nyloned foot.

"Yes, I can," he replied, and pulled a revolver out of his jacket pocket. He raised it, aiming it straight at my face.

For a brief moment, I stared at the gun. At the perfect round hole at the end of the barrel. Then I reached and grasped his other arm. Jerked him inside. "You come with me." I pulled him down the narrow hallway that ran to the left of the front door. Past the guest bathroom. Past the niche in the wall that held the shiny black telephone it had taken two years to get installed. Through the dining room with the lacquered long table and the glass-fronted cabinet glittering with silver and china and crystal. I hauled him into the pantry section of the kitchen. "Stay here!" I ordered, and whipped around the wall that separated the pantry from the rest of the kitchen. "Go!" I commanded the two servants working there. They rushed off down the short hall that led to their rooms.

My friend stood where I'd left him, the gun still in his hand. I ignored the gun and gave a little jump and plopped myself atop one of the counters, beside the straw basket holding avocadoes and limes and long-pointed chiles. From this higher vantage point, I wagged a finger at him. "And just what do you think you're doing?"

"That music's too loud."

The music *was* loud. He took a step and closed the space between us. The gun barrel was now level with my mouth. It was perhaps a foot away from my lips.

I held his gaze. He was sweating. Beads of perspiration had turned his hair into baby curls.

"You're sweating," I said, reaching out to touch his cheek. His eyes were wild.

He lifted a hand and batted my hand away. He swiped the sweat in his eyes with a finger. "Esa música . . . "

I made that same explosive little sound nana used to make to show her irritation. I hopped off the counter. "Wait here." I strode purposely into the living room. My friends were still on the patio, writhing to the throb of the music. I went over to the stereo and turned the music down.

Back in the pantry, my friend still held the gun. I pulled myself back upon the counter. "Aren't you going to put that thing away?" I asked.

"Why should I?"

"Because I want you to."

"That's not a good reason."

"Okay then, because I turned the music down."

His eyes narrowed as if he were mulling the fact over.

In the room, the only sound was the hum of the refrigerator's motor. It was a GE, a 1928 model, fueled by kerosene. "You asked me to turn down the music and I did, didn't I?"

"You did."

"So then put the gun away."

He said nothing, but lowered the gun to his side.

I climbed down from the counter and stood beside him. I laid a hand gently on his arm. "Please put the gun away." Softly I said this.

He slipped the gun into his jacket pocket. "It was the music," he muttered.

"I know." I led him from the room, past the dining room and the telephone niche and the bathroom and into the foyer. I opened the door and he stepped out onto the driveway. His opened hand was spread over his pocket.

"You can go home now."

"Vaya pues." Okay then. He turned away from me.

I closed the door and locked it. I went back to the stereo. With a quick turn of the wrist, I cranked the music back up. On the patio, I smiled at Jay, lifting my arms to the furious rhythm of a new song.

I mentioned earlier I could be ugly, but my God, what an imbecile I'd been. Thinking back, I couldn't say if the gun was loaded or not. It doesn't matter. What matters is that I'm very sure it was that day when alcohol and me began our close relationship. Alcohol lifted me from the confounding realities of my life. Alcohol emboldened me and turned me rash. Alcohol allowed me to be someone I was not.

• • •

In Missouri, high school ended a year later. After one last summer spent at home in El Salvador, I'd be entering college in the fall. But that May night in Unionville, on the eve of my departure, I strolled out past the barn and stood at the edge of the pasture, beyond the brightness of the barn light. That afternoon, I had wept and hugged my friends goodbye. Shari, Darlene, Judy, Betty, Joyce, Alice. Off I'd go and leave them behind. I looked out across the darkened fields, feeling the curtain of that theater inside me lowering itself again to the stage floor. Another act over. Soon, the curtain would rise to yet another reality. How different it would be from the one I had been living, I could only guess.

I turned back toward the house sitting stern and silent against the night sky. Light burning back in the kitchen formed an uncertain glow around the front windows. I thought, in this world you make connections where you can, and started toward the light.

• • •

In the morning, the day broke clear and sunny. A perfect day for an airplane ride. Grandpa had filled up the '49 Dodge at the gas pump he had rigged from an oil drum on a platform and a hose. The Dodge was nine years old. It was olive drab and the steering wheel was ebony and very shiny, dulled only at the ten and two spots by contact with grandpa's calloused hands. Grandpa was driving me down the interstate, to the airport, which was three hours away, in Kansas City. I was wearing a new suit grandma had made. These were the late fifties, when flying was a grand occasion that merited dressing up. My suit was fashioned of black faille and featured a straight skirt and a bolero jacket. I had picked the pattern and fabric myself, much to grandma's consternation. "Oh, honey," she said when I spilled my purchases from the bag onto the kitchen table. "This'll make up gloomy. A girl like you needs something cheery." Grandma had marched me over to the chifforobe stuffed with folded lengths of fabric, some saved from flour sacks she'd bought at the Hy-Vee. I shook my head and would not be swayed. "I must have black," I said, not bothering to explain that, in Salvador, life was a formal affair shaped by unquestioned protocol: During the day, I wore colored dresses and skirts. After five and on important occasions, such as flying, it was dark clothing I had to wear. Going home, I would leave behind my blue jeans and sweatshirts, my bobby sox and tennis shoes.

Grandpa revved up the Dodge and we pulled away from the old house and rolled down the gravel driveway that led past the new house and to the road. Grandma rode along too. She was in the front seat and because we were heading for the big city, she wore the pastel duster she'd made herself for Easter. A squat hat with a pink feather sat squarely on her head. Grandpa had on striped overalls so clean they were stiff and smelled heavily of lye. In deference to the occasion, he wore a white shirt and a patterned tie, two more things grandma had made at her Singer.

In the back seat, I looked out the window and mouthed a goodbye to Fido, grandpa's German shepherd, who stood at the edge of the yard and was too old to want to come along. I mouthed a goodbye to the outhouse and the bunkhouse, to the chicken house and the corncrib, to the sheep shed and the barn. When we drove by, the milk cows stood reluctantly in the barnyard and I waved to Bossie, who was always cranky and who liked to stamp a leg when grandma milked her. I waved to the cluster of speckled hens scurrying out of the car's way, to the flock of ewes and their lambs grazing way off in the pasture.

Though I'd flown home for summers past, I'd lived in these surroundings for three years. I did not know it then, but after time I'd come to understand that in El Salvador, life was frail and most always capricious, that people found joy in the midst of insurmountable obstacles, that in the end, it is hope that saves us. I'd learn, too, that in Missouri, life was what you make of it, that satisfaction comes with a job well done, that in the end, it is steadfastness that sustains us.

But back then these thoughts had yet to strike me.

Back then, with my high school days behind me, I was at the farm, in the green Dodge, heading down the road that joined one of my worlds to the other. I ran a hand over the car's tuck and roll upholstery. In the crease between the top and back of the seat, a slender leaf of corn poked out. I gave it a pull and it resisted and I realized the corn was growing there. This was not an uncommon thing. Frequently grandpa hauled corn to town in the Dodge. I imagined a handful of corn spilling out from a sack. Imagined one of the kernels taking root a world away from the field. Any living thing could do this. If we're adaptable, we can thrive and bloom in foreign soil.

• • •

To enter college, I didn't have to go far. Northeast Missouri State Teachers' College at Kirksville (now Truman State University) was an hour away from the farm. In 1959, I enrolled and moved into the dorm. The summer before, while home in El Salvador on vacation, I'd had a talk with Daddy. I wanted to be a doctor, I told him, but he dissuaded me from the idea, pointing out that for a girl, a teaching career would be a wiser choice. An obedient daughter, I did as he suggested, and studied for a B.S. degree in secondary education. Gregarious and extroverted, I threw myself into college life. I dated (just like Archie and Veronica!), joined a sorority, was on the cheerleading squad, and, when I was a sophomore, was even elected Homecoming Queen. Not resting on my laurels, I belonged to a number of campus organizations, including the drama club, starring in a few campus productions because of it. Despite the hoopla, I didn't neglect my studies. In fact, I graduated *cum laude.* All this to say, that while I was working hard, while I was a whirling dervish and thoroughly enjoying being one, my gut was pitching a fit. Once again the stomachaches, the bloating, the dramatic swings between diarrhea and constipation. I tried laxatives, of course, but they often caused cramps so severe that I was reluctant to keep using them.

When I was a junior, I had frequent dates with a young man from Tenafly, New Jersey, who was studying at the College of Osteopathic Medicine—Kirksville being the birthplace of this often misunderstood branch of science. As I recall, his name was Harry. I remember his curly hair, his dark, brooding good-looks. Harry was hell-bent on being a doctor, which thrilled me, given my secret yearning to be one as well. While other couples grabbed a meal, or took in a movie, Harry would sneak me into the dissecting room, the place with the stainless-steel tables and the draped corpses lying like sacrifices upon them. Harry would lead me to his own special table, to his own special cadaver. He'd respectfully pull back the drape and make his introduction. "Hello, Rosie, this is Sandy," he would say at every meeting, and I'd hold my breath against the overwhelming odor of formalin that helped preserve the generous Rosie who had made herself available for such extraordinary use. She had been an old woman when she died. She lay there, her long slender body leathery and browned by the preservative. Harry would give a little lecture about whatever it was that he was studying at the time. Lost in reverence and wonder, Harry'd wax on about the muscles and fasciae that lay like crisscrossed bands under the bony cage of Rosie's ribs. Before leaving, Harry would relocate the drape. "You're a grand old gal, Rosie," he'd say before we turned away.

Compassionate, Harry was, intuitive and caring. One time, when we were having coffee, noting that I'd barely touched my caramel roll, he asked what was the matter. "Oh, nothing," I said. How do you tell a date that you hadn't, except for what my sister likes to call *las insignificantes bolitas* (the insignificant little balls), had a bowel movement in over a week? "I'm okay." I must say here that there was no undercurrent of a possible sexual complication, like an accidental pregnancy. Harry and I were simply friends. We had smooched a time or two, but our passion was not for each other, but for the awesome institution of medicine. For Rosie and for all she could impart.

"You look pretty pale to me."

"I might be a little pale." That old lethargy had come back. It was a struggle to drag myself out of bed to climb the ever-higher mountain of perfectionism I was making of my life.

"I should take a look at that." Harry dug into his caramel roll, a roll so large it fell over the side of the plate.

"Take a look at what?"

"Your blood, silly."

And so I let Harry take a look at my blood.

It was not an easy thing. It wasn't as if Harry were a licensed doctor and I could make an appointment and he could, in a clinic somewhere, draw blood into a syringe and then take it to the lab. He was a mere medical student—albeit one in his sophomore year—and as such it was most certainly against the law for him to be digging around for a vein in my arm.

I've never forgotten the night of the digging. It was late March, as I recall. One of those chilly, foggy nights right out of "The Hound of the Baskervilles." As if this were a drug deal or an abortion we were about to undertake, we were leery and cautious. He had had to filch the proper equipment from medical school: a big fat syringe, an assortment of needles, that little rubber tube he'd tie around my arm. The vial that would hold my blood. I remember that we'd been scheduled to use a friend's house, but when we arrived, we'd been hurried off to another location. I, of course, was terrified. I had never before experienced this procedure—that's what Harry called it, a "procedure." At nineteen, I was a blood-giving virgin.

It turned out that Harry was a blood-taking one.

The procedure started out well enough. Harry was all serious intent; he was, after all, actually playing doctor. He sat me down at a desk in a room. He rolled up the sleeve of my big purple sweatshirt (KSTC BULLDOGS!), straightened out my arm and propped it on the desktop, under a lamp with a broad glass shade. Gravely, he studied the network of veins spidered under my flesh, then tied the rubber ligature around the top of my arm. He swabbed me thoroughly with alcohol, then flicked a bent finger against the crook of my arm. "Make a fist," he said, and I did, turning away from the sight of my arm, the needle, from Harry himself, so determined and focused. I tried to distract myself by looking about the room, a small space at the top of a flight of stairs, the runners of which had creaked as we'd hurried up them. The walls slanted, as they had in my room at the farm. A dresser against a wall. Missing pulls on a few drawers. A narrow lumpy bed with a ribbed olive-green spread.

Near me, scattered on the desk, books, papers, notepads. A coffee cup. Old, film-topped coffee half filling it.

It was not going well for Harry. He couldn't find a vein. He couldn't puncture any vein he did find. Little beads of sweat had popped out across his brow. His needle was a gouge, as he pricked and poked. "Your veins are slippery," he said, almost to himself. "They keep rolling over." The image of such a thing caused the room to tilt a bit, caused a little buzz to start up in my ears. The pain he was inflicting brought tears to my eyes, but I bit my lip and struggled to be brave as he continued digging. When the ordeal was finally over, when my bright red blood filled the vial he'd brought along, and he'd taped cotton-balls over the excavation sites, the room swam in earnest. I said, "I think I'm going to faint."

Harry pressed my head down between my legs. "Take deep breaths," he said, keeping a gentle pressure on the back of my neck. When I tried to stand, I felt my legs go to rubber and Harry walked me to the bed, laid me down. "I'll get you some juice," he said, and I heard his every step as he rushed down the stairs and then back up them again.

Empty juice glass on the desk, Harry settled down beside me. The feel of his shoulder, his hip against me, was a sweet tender thing and I began silently to cry. I cried for the ache in my arm and for the ache in my heart. Hot tears slipped down my cheeks and pooled in my ears at the thought of my condition. I was a motherless child, far away from home, lying in an attic garret, my crazy-mixed-up life swirling like a maelstrom around me. I was sad, so sad, so filled up, so constipated. Harry snuggled an arm under my neck and I laid my head upon his chest, and took in his woodsy, sweaty smell. As I'd done in nana's laundry room, I slipped my thumb into my mouth, and for close to an hour, I sobbed so hard my tears soaked the front of his sweatshirt, the sleeve of mine. I sobbed so hard my nose clogged and I had to open my mouth wide to pop the vacuum in my ears. Harry said nothing. He just lay there and listened.

It was so like me, keeping my sad self hidden from those who really mattered: my parents, grandparents, my sister and friends. Folks who might have rejected my vulnerability, might have even rejected *me,* had they known my true feelings. Or so I believed. And why not? Hadn't I been sent away? For a good reason, perhaps, and to family, but still, if I allowed myself the truth, it sometimes felt like banishment. God knows I worked hard, wherever I found myself, at being a perfect and happy girl, but every now and then . . . well, my blue skies clouded up, and with people like nana and Harry, with people like them I felt I could risk a downpour. Just a little bitty one.

That night, when Harry and I left the attic room, I held on to his arm all the way to the dorm. All the time, keenly aware of the little vial of blood he carried in his pocket.

A week later, after the dark angry bruises had paled from my arm, I was hospitalized. Enemas were given to relieve colon impaction. Harry stayed away, given I'd delivered myself into someone else's care. My blood had gone untested, it seemed, for the same reason.

A few months later, on my way home to El Salvador for summer vacation, I made a stop in New Orleans, where my aunt and uncle and my cousins lived. My parents had arranged that I be examined at the Ochner Clinic, for my hospitalization in Kirksville had worried them.

At the clinic, the doctor listened to my litany of complaints: constipation, the diarrhea, etc. His pronouncement was that I had "a nervous stomach." Still, he took a sample of my blood, a quick, painless procedure this time. When the results of the blood test came in, he discovered that what had caused my gut problem was a nasty infestation of intestinal parasites: Nematodes to be exact. They sent me home with pills so large they looked like something grandpa sometimes forced down a Guernsey's throat when it got the bloat.

That summer, I spent the first week of my vacation choking down pills, pooping out whip worms.

• • •

Thankfully, the following years were quiet ones as far as my gut was concerned. My life, however, continued as active as ever. In fact, in my junior year, I fell in love.

He was tall and slender, a year older than I, but just a freshman. A late bloomer when it came to education. I'd see him frequently in the lobby of my dorm, sitting under the starry chandelier at the grand piano. He filled the space with music: ragtime, jazz, rock. His repertoire seemed never-ending. When he began to add his own tunes, began to sing his own catchy lyrics, a ring of coeds circling the piano, I'd often pause and watch him. Watch him sway to the music, his long fingers flying up and down the keyboard.

It happened that I was running for Student Council that year, and there were posters all over campus with my name and picture on them. One evening, there came a call for me, and I hurried down the dorm hall to the phone.

It was a man's voice, a voice vaguely familiar. "I've seen you all over the place on those posters. When I'm at the piano in your dorm, I've caught you watching me."

And so it began. Dates for coffee and the movies. Long walks under the campus trees. Drives in the country. Intimacies in the front seat. Everything we did, punctuated by music, for in addition to the piano, he played the guitar, and soon I learned his songs and we would harmonize.

• • •

A year later, although he had quit college to return to Saint Louis and work, we were engaged. Up north in Kirksville, where we would marry, I waited out the weeks before graduation and our wedding day. One mid-fall evening, strolling up a street to my dorm, I kicked amber-leaves, my breath feathery before me. The air was heady with the smell of smoke curling lazily from fireplace chimneys. I passed houses with wide steps and deep porches displaying lighted jack-o'-lanterns with silly grins. I passed windows radiant in the yellow wash of just-turned-on lights. I thought, this is how my life can be: a sheltered street, a welcoming house with home fires burning. In one house, I spotted a woman gazing dreamily out into the evening, her hands busy at something the window frame kept me from observing. In a backyard, children caroused and tumbled in a pile of fallen leaves. I continued on, thinking that at this time of day it was only women and children who made up the world. Where are the men? I asked myself, and thought of my own man. How we'd soon marry. How with him I might begin to really open up. How together we'd create all the home I'd ever need.

• • •

After I graduated college, we married and I moved to Saint Louis and started teaching high-school English and Spanish. Within two years' time, my husband and I had two baby boys, Christopher and Jonathon. Big, round babies with peach-colored cheeks and fat tiny fists. I nursed them both in an old red rocker, looking down into their sweet, somber faces. I sang them each the same lilting tune: *Where are you going, my little one, little one? Where are you going, my baby, my own?*

Back then, only sunny skies. No dark clouds on my horizon.

• • •

While pregnant with Jon, I'd gained a lot of weight and my bowel problems started up again. That little bump I'd discovered when I was eight came back with a vengeance. I'll spare you the unpleasant details, but suffice it to say that after years of agony, I ended up in surgery. Hemorrhoidectomies are not pleasant experiences. They are so low on the scale of surgeries-to-brag-about that having one is a very lonely, and very painful, experience. I had mine in the late sixties. Thirty-plus years later, I trust there's been improvement in that area.

When I was in the hospital, I shared a room with a nameless young woman who insisted that the curtain that separated the beds, and which most people ignore, be pulled shut. For the three days I was hospitalized, my roommate was but a disembodied voice behind the curtain. She moaned, she sobbed, and when I threw my own voice up over the drape to ask if I might help, she sobbed even louder.

One night, when I'd been soundly asleep, I was awakened by lights and voices and something going on over there. Our nurse was saying, "It's okay. It's okay." My roommate, "Oh no, oh no, oh no." A fecal smell, but with a sickly sweet edge, wafted my way. I thought, Oh God, that poor thing! The voices continued. Hers, "I'll never get the hang of it. Never. It'll never stay on." Our nurse's, "Of course you will. You just have to get used to it."

Lying in bed, my bottom packed in gauze and throbbing, I tried to decipher what was being said. My half of the room was shrouded in shadow, and all these goings-on seemed largely important and enigmatic. What are they talking about? I asked myself. What in heaven's name is going on over there?

Early in the morning, before the nurse went off duty, she came in for a quick check. In a whisper, I asked her what had happened during the night.

"Oh, Julie's bag broke," she replied.

"Oh," I said, nodding as if I understood.

Julie, the name was. The voice beyond the drape was Julie's. But what was that about a bag? What kind of bag was that? I could not begin to imagine.

• • •

About this time, it dawned on me that I had a chronic problem. Though weeks, months even, could go by without a symptom or complaint, soon enough, the tide would turn and I'd be back in the soup again. To make matters worse, my marriage was starting to unravel.

One spring, perhaps as recreational therapy, my husband and I decided to get away for a few days. We flew to New Orleans, a place that held dear memories because of the times I'd stopped there on my way home to El Salvador. We stayed in the French Quarter, at one of those quaint establishments you spy as you stroll down a cobbled street. Ours was a romantic B&B that loomed behind a curlicued iron gate. Our room was off a fragrant patio with its own gurgling fountain. We feasted at Antoine's (the oysters Rockefeller, no spinach in their recipe!), breakfasted at Brennan's (the café Brulot, the Eggs Sardou) and, at the Café du Monde, enjoyed thick chicory coffee and beignets (confectioner's sugar everywhere). Staying in the Quarter was to be enveloped in sensuality: the joyful soulful melodies floating out of bistros, the barkers attempting to lure you into neon-lighted strip joints, the scent of jasmine riding on the velvety night air. And with it all, lingering on our tongues, the taste of Ramos Gin Fizzes, of mint juleps, the little fires they lit in our hearts and south of our hearts.

One night, we'd had dinner, and we were mellow mellow, when the urge to use the toilet hit me so strongly, I had to steady myself against the wall of a building. To be sure there were bathrooms nearby, one in every establishment that surrounded us, but I couldn't bear the thought of using such a public place. My husband in tow, I lurched and stumbled toward our inn, pain knotting my gut as I concentrated with all my might on holding it, holding it.

Reaching our bathroom, I was a mad woman throwing off shoes, peeling off hose, bra, panties, slip, dress. A clammy perspiration dampened my face, neck, breasts. I flung up the toilet seat and plunked myself down, the pain doubling me. My husband stood in the doorway, looking helpless. "Go, go, go," I said, motioning for him to go out the door and sit in the patio. Sourness filled my mouth. My body was so sensitive that the pressure of earrings, bracelet, wedding bands was excruciating. I pulled these off too, laid them at my bare feet. Soon the narrow little room filled with that same sickly sweet odor that had wafted up over the hospital curtain when, years before, Julie's bag had broken.

As I did the night that Harry from New Jersey had lain beside me listening, I propped my head against the wall and sobbed. I sobbed for my crumbling marriage, for the future of my precious boys, for my own vulnerable body. I sobbed for how alone I felt in this grief, for as was my way, I had not breathed a word of my situation to my family.

• • •

I decided to switch doctors. I'd been seeing a general practitioner, and while he had been of much use, I thought that a colon and rectal specialist would serve me better. I found one at a clinic close to home.

On my first visit, I laid out for him my list of maladies: fierce cramping, weight loss, the dramatic swings between diarrhea and constipation, the rectal bleeding now, the mucous in the stool, that awful urge to defecate that would frequently beset me. He scheduled me for a sigmoidoscopy, a look-see with a lighted scope up the rectum and along the sigmoid, the last ten centimeters of the descending colon. To prepare for the exam, the colon needed to be emptied and thoroughly cleaned, and so began my long acquaintanceship with all manner of enemas and with awful-tasting purgatives. This was in the days before the flexible scope and when, for the exam, you had to kneel and lay the top half of yourself across a short table that was then tilted so that your business-end could be attended to. No matter how well the nurse draped you, no matter how breezy her repartee before the procedure (that word again), it was still a humiliating experience to know that your naked butt was poking straight up there, the doctor's big lamp shining down on it like a spotlight.

I know it's an oft-told medical tale, but it actually happened to me that on that first visit, when my colon was as clean as the legendary whistle, when the doctor began his examination, he came upon something so curious? so astonishing? so rare?, that he asked my pardon and left the room for a moment, returning with a colleague whom he introduced to me as I lay bent over the table, my backside high above my head. My face burning, I mumbled a hello to a white-coated torso, to black shiny shoes, the only part of the visitor I could spy.

The doctor continued with his examination, making comments to the torso as he inched the probe, very painfully I must say, along the inside of my gut. "See that?" A pause. "Looks pretty grainy." Another pause. "Here, too, don't you think?"

What they saw was inflamed and raw and red. What they saw was an active case of inflammatory bowel disease. Ulcerative colitis, to put a proper name on it.

• • •

Until now, I've left out my concern with personal cleanliness, but I'll go into it, because after the diagnosis, what had been fastidiousness became an obsession. For better or for worse, I must implicate my mother in this. Where it concerned the nether-parts, she was the queen of clean. "Make sure you wipe. Wipe really well," she used to say. Early on, she offered a tip. "After you're through, moisten the paper with water. That will help get you clean."

Of course, I took her advice, but multiplied it to the nth power. One, two, three turns of TP over the wrist. Wad the paper up. Reach over to the faucet (it mattered very much the proximity of sink and toilet), run the paper quickly through the water, then wipe, wipe, wipe for cleanliness. Drop the wad into the toilet. Finish off with a few more sheets, then pat, pat, pat for dryness. Needless to say, over the years, we're talking lots and lots of Charmin here. In addition to that, mountains of Tucks, those wonderful moist towelettes.

I think back to the farm and the family's dream house grandpa built by the side of the road. A house with central heating. With running water from the newly dug well. A house with a bathroom that contained a toilet, sink and bathtub. I lived in that house for my last two years of high school, totally relieved that using the outhouse was a thing of the past. (Still, old customs die hard. Despite the spankingly modern inside bathroom, grandma had grandpa build her a new outhouse out in the back. For old times' sake, she liked to go out there at times and make use of the facilities.)

Though the new bathroom had been a blessing, something, somehow had gone wrong with the toilet's waste pipe. Some sort of poor connection, so that when you flushed, more often than not, the paper clogged, and, horror of horrors, the waters climbed. To complicate matters, because we used a well, it appeared that the pressure was at times inadequate to swish the paper down and away. In any case, because of the problem, a trash can had been placed beside the toilet. All—ALL, get it?—toilet paper would be deposited in that. I'll spare you the details concerning the pros and cons of the new system. Suffice it to say, I had gone back to "holding it."

Of course, this kind of manipulation of body functions is not good for what ails you. In fact, sometimes it's the very cause of what ails you.

• • •

Married with children in Saint Louis, I started going a little nuts. Chronic illness and a rocky marriage will sometimes do that to a gal. I remember one time in particular. I was at the stove, making dinner when the phone rang. A woman was on the line. A woman who took in a breath and then quickly hung up. Back then, spinning in the vortex of my marital storm, I was certain I was crazy. When my husband came home and we'd had a quick cocktail, when the four of us were sitting down to eat, that phone call filled up my head again. Recalling the woman's swift intake of breath sent me over the edge. I picked up the steaming roast I'd made and heaved it, football-style. Oh, my, but I'm neurotic, I thought, as it sailed across the kitchen and thunked the wall above the stove. On to the green beans, these thrown in fistfuls against the window overlooking the kids' sandbox. I plucked up the rolls and sent little buttered missiles flying. Then I spied the gravy bowl. I dipped a hand in and flung. Arcs of brown gravy hung for milliseconds in the air before splatting against pictures and cabinets, the cookie jar and pans. Gee, but I'm crazy, I thought. Splat. Oh, but I'm sick. Splat. God, but I'm sick and crazy. Splat. Splat. Splat.

• • •

Of course, I *was* ill, and there were crazy-making medications for my illness. A diagnosis of inflammatory bowel disease brings with it an obligatory familiarity with the drugs used to treat it. In my case, the doctor put me immediately on two forms of remedy: Azulfidine, the trade name for *sulfasalizine,* and Cortenemas, hydrocortisone retention enemas.

Azulfidine has been used for over fifty years, and usually it was the first and preferred medication used to treat bowel inflammation. Now, years later, newer drugs have supplanted it, but back then, the doctor prescribed two grams of Azulfidine or four tablets a day. It wasn't long before the side-effects kicked in: headache, nausea, especially the nausea. You would've thought that I was newly pregnant, the nausea was so bad, but what could I do? Because of the drug, the inflammation was subsiding and with it my symptoms: the terrible *tenesmus,* that urgent push that makes you think you have to go, the bloody stools, the mucous passed because of the sloughing off of the colon lining, so compared to all these, nausea and headache were a piece of cake. (Not really, but you get the idea.) And so I bit my lip and suffered through. Fortunately, not long after, a coated form of the tablets came on the market and these released the drug more slowly into the small intestine. This proved to be the answer to the pesky side-effects.

The Cortenemas, however, were another matter entirely. These, while extremely cute in their mini-plastic, 100mg bottles with their long and flashy turquoise tips, well, with these, there was nothing to do but grin and bare it. Grin and bear it, as well. My prescribed treatment called for morning and nightly applications. We're talking *retention* here, as in squeeze the liquid in, and then don't let the liquid out. For it to be useful, the medication needs to be fully absorbed by rectal tissue. Sometimes this could take up to an hour.

For me, enema-taking involved concentration. I'll pass along my method, in hope it might be helpful: Pick a private place where you won't be disturbed. In the bathroom, on a fluffy rug and towel. Or on the bed, this too overspread with a towel. Put on some soothing music. "The Memory of Trees" by Enya would be nice. Lay on your left side. Breathe deeply. Squeeze the liquid out bit by bit. Slow administration will shortcut that awful need to evacuate, so take your time. Don't be rushed. All the while entertain wondrous thoughts of this miraculous drug prednisone, how it's bathing and healing your poor aching butt.

Needless to say, my history of "holding it" proved to be a real bonus where retention enemas were concerned.

• • •

In the early seventies, I became a stay-at-home mom. I'd recently received an MA in Education and Comparative Literature and our family of four had moved from Missouri to Minnesota. We lived in the suburbs of Minneapolis, out in Mound, on a huge multi-bayed lake called Minnetonka. Chris and Jon were twelve and ten.

My husband, now a successful songwriter by trade, worked for an incentives company. He wrote music and lyrics for trade shows and business incentive programs. Since moving from Missouri, I had searched for a teaching job, but there was a glut of teachers all over the country, so I was forced to stay home. Having the time, I began to write.

Other than for newsy letters, I'd never really written before. It never occurred to me that I might be a storyteller. My father was a marvelous raconteur, often regaling us and his friends with accounts of his exploits: growing up on the farm, both in Missouri and then Idaho, joining the Navy at 18, being appointed to Annapolis, working as a page in the Senate in Washington, meeting Martita Benítez, the love of his life, their living in Mexico and then El Salvador. My darling Daddy. He could go on and on.

My own storytelling efforts began with writing little personal scenes. When I began to put words on paper, I found that I was much like Daddy. To help keep focused, I joined a writer's group and soon began filling a few notebooks. After much encouragement from the instructor and my fellow classmates, I decided to write a novel. Seemed like a natural progression. No matter that novel-writing was as mysterious to me as what lay under the sea. I'll learn by doing, I thought, and started a book set in Missouri. On, surprise, surprise!, a Missouri farm. A sort of mystery about a young girl who witnesses a murder and who is pursued by the murderer as she tries to bring him to justice.

I found that writing was uplifting both to my sensibilities and, in a metaphysical kind of way, to my gut. I'd sit at my clunky typewriter in a room with a view of the lake and the writing would transport me. I'd be lost in story, forgetting for a time how seriously in trouble my marriage was, forgetting how sick I could be.

About that time, an unexpected job opportunity popped up. Wilson Learning Corporation, a sales and management training company, needed a translator on a freelance basis. They had a program for Canadian bank personnel that consisted of a leader's guide, various study guides, audio cassettes and, in those days before video, film strips. The bank had offices in the Dominican Republic and needed the program in Spanish. Because I was bilingual, and had lived for many years in Latin America, I was hired by the director of the international department for the job. The director's name was Jim Kondrick.

The work paid well, and it was fulfilling. I could translate at home, in my room with the lake views, and so I set the novel aside, promising myself that when the time was right, I'd get back to it.

Oh that I could have set aside my illness as easily. But no. The flare-ups came and went. When they hit me, I kept the news to myself, because an illness like ulcerative colitis is not exactly a fashionable topic of conversation; it is an unmentionable illness. Given the symptoms, an illness to hide.

To illustrate the point, I remember the summer of '76. Chris and Jon were about to go off to Missouri to visit their paternal grandparents for an extended stay at their sprawling country place, a place the family called "the farm." A few days before they left, we planned an all-day trip to Afton, Minnesota, where we would float on inner tubes down the Apple River. It's a popular pastime, for despite Minnesota's reputation for cold weather, the summers are often hot and sticky, and floating for two hours down a cool, meandering stream is the definition of bliss.

Chris and Jon were ecstatic about our coming adventure. We'd be going with two other couples. The eight of us would drive to the put-in place, where we'd rent large inner tubes, the kind that come from tractors. Like those gigantic ones on Daddy's Caterpillars. The plan was to float idly down the river, trailing an extra inner tube that would hold a small cooler with refreshments. At the take-out point, we'd board a bus that would return us to our cars.

Two days before the big adventure, I had a relapse that had me surreptitiously scooting in and out of our only bathroom, dousing the place with air freshener after its use, putting on a happy face when my boys would study me, their expressions somber, their eyes filled with questions: Are you sick again, Mom? Are we still going to go? Do we have to stay home?

Well, of course, we were going to go. We were all going to go.

As I remember, on the day we went, the weather cooperated splendidly. Blue sky, fluffy clouds. The river lazy and wide. We'd all slathered on sunscreen; in addition to our swimsuits, we'd donned caps with long bills and wore tennis shoes, a must for careening down the rocky rapids at the end of the float. The rapids consisted of a series of step-downs in the riverbed over which the water tumbled fast and frothy. As if they'd soon be riding the roller coaster at Six Flags, all week long, Chris and Jon had babbled about shooting the Apple River rapids in their inner tubes. They planned to do it many times, for we'd learned that after going over, you could walk back up the bank and shoot down again. As we floated, they kept up a patter about what lay ahead, our friends egging them on, they themselves looking forward to the plunge.

Not me. I took the trip, a smile plastered on my face, chattering inanely, my mind churning with the effort to keep my rear-gates shut, sealed, locked up. Though we were on a river, and millions of cubic meters were flowing under us, the thought of letting go and polluting was as unsavory as peeing in a swimming pool.

When we neared the rapids, I took charge of the inner tube with the refreshments, and pulled it up onto the bank. I found a nice shallow spot in the water, and sat myself down between two smooth stones, my arms propped up.

"Watch me, Mom, watch," my boys yelled out and I'd raise a hand and give a wave. Called out encouragement as they trudged back up to plunge down again.

Soon, it was no use, my inner fortitude collapsed and I had to let go. Let go into the river. I sat there for close to an hour trying with all my might to disconnect from what I had no power to control. I watched my sons, their browned and glistening supple bodies, their gleefulness, their pure and tender hearts.

Tears joined the perspiration sliding down my face. That terrible dread was at my doorstep again: something dark and unfathomable was looming just around life's corner.

• • •

After the boys left for the farm, I threw myself into the translation work. Because the deadline was fast approaching, I made frequent trips to Wilson Learning, where Jim Kondrick and I conferred over the text. Often, we'd go to lunch. Over time and over beers, we started sharing our personal lives. Though I was not totally direct and neither was he, it soon became apparent that we were both unhappily married. As far as my illness was concerned, I said not a word of this to him.

On August 6, 1976, my husband and I, plus our dear friend Ed Bock, who had recently moved to the Twin Cities from Saint Louis, were invited to a party at a house also on the lake. I tried begging off. As usual, I did not feel well, but this I did not admit (that old embarrassment, again). I just said I needed to keep working. The translation deadline was less than a week away. But Eddie and my husband cajoled me into going.

The party was in full swing when we arrived. Guests, drinks in hand, lolled in the living room and around the big island in the kitchen where our hostess was slapping out hamburger patties and stacking them on a tray. There were guests out on the wide deck that overlooked the lake. On the deck sat the grill. Under its lid, foil-wrapped potatoes and corn were already roasting.

I made myself a gin and tonic. For the past few years, I'd been drinking more than usual. I was not alone in this. These were, after all, the seventies, when, at parties, all manner of libations were abundant. I remember how it was back then. Cocktails before dinner. Wine with dinner. Dessert drinks or cordials after dinner. While our group had not taken to drugs or grass as so many of our generation had, it was alcohol that satisfied us, that fired us up. Generally, in the winter, it was martinis. Gin and tonics in the summer. At all times, red, white or rosé wine. And not to leave out the ice-cream drinks made with anything called "crème"—crème de menthe, crème de cacao, crème de who-knows-what-else.

As for me, I accepted with gratitude every single drink offered me. Thirstily, I drank every single drink down. Drank it down hastily, my arm extended for another. Drinking eased the pain in my gut and in my butt.

Drinking eased the pain in my life.

But drinking also screwed up my head. With booze warming me, my people-pleasing, easygoing, compliant self fell away. I'd grow bold and loud and contrary. I was doing it that day at the party. I was in the kitchen, and my husband was holding court in the living room. He was talking about a recent business trip he'd taken to Spain. He was talking about some señorita. My husband, the songwriter, was talking about the song he'd written about the señorita. Something about how she was for hire. About how a man has to do what he has to do. He began to sing the song.

I think I hurled a glass at him. Maybe even my gin and tonic. Because of the gin already clouding my brain, these events seem rather fuzzy. But I'm certain I made a scene. A bit of screaming and yelling. A bit of threatening. Maybe even a bit of swatting. As in, lashing out with a hand and trying to kill the son of a bitch.

I think it was Eddie who tried calming me. Eddie who took me gently by the hand and escorted me out onto the deck where our host had now retreated to begin to casually flip the burgers. It was only the three of us on the deck; the rest of the guests were perhaps huddling inside.

I gulped down the evening air. Beyond the deck, jutting some fifteen feet above the lawn that rolled down toward the lake, the sun was setting over the water. The firmament was wild with pinks and crimsons, and I felt the flame of the same coloring in my cheeks. Holy God, I was making such a mess of things.

Eddie and I walked over to the railing. I gave a long sigh and turned to look at him. "Shit," I think I said. I think he smiled ruefully, for he was, and still is, the kind of friend who never stands in judgment. I think I might have smiled back. What I *do* know is that I turned. Turned to lean back against the railing. Eddie did it, too. A moment later, there came the awful sound of nails pulling out of wood. Like fingernails against a blackboard, a short high screech before the railing broke free.

Eddie and I. We dropped backward into space.

• • •

What you learn when you fall from a high deck is that inflammatory bowel disease pales in comparison.

Eddie and I fell hard, fortuitously, against grass-covered ground. I can still recall that horrifying weightlessness seconds after the plummet, that stupefying contact with land, back first, then head, and finally feet, all in a whiplash effect. We lay crumpled there, Eddie and I, and there were sounds coming from both of us that were positively inhuman. The guttural wrenching sounds you make when all the air has gone out of your lungs, when there seems to be no air whatsoever left in the world.

Needless to say, the accident shut the party down. An ambulance was quickly summoned, guests scurried about, someone said something about Eddie and I being moved. This I vividly remember, as I remember croaking out "Don't move me. Don't anybody touch me."

Except for the paramedics who soon slipped a board under me for transportation, it's a good thing no one did. Later, it would be discovered that I'd suffered three shattered vertebrae, the shards of which were lying menacingly against the spinal cord. One small wrong movement and, Slice! I'd become a paraplegic.

Eddie and I were rushed, siren wailing, to a nearby regional hospital where we were X-rayed. I remember my husband bending over me after getting the results. He whispered, "Your back is broken. They're transferring you to Minneapolis. This place can't handle broken backs." Years later, he would reveal how near he was to leaving me that night. It was the accident, he said, that kept him from getting into his car and driving to the airport, where he was going to fly off. To where, I'll never know.

Eddie's injuries, while as painful as mine, were not as limb- or life-threatening. He was not hospitalized that night, but given the pain he's endured over the years, it's now evident that he should have been.

In a second ambulance, on the way to St. Mary's Hospital in Minneapolis, I went into shock and it was like a curtain dropping down before me.

Only snatches of memory remain concerning that first week in the intensive care unit. I was in critical condition, hooked up to monitors that whirred on and clicked off. Only these small soft sounds to let me know I was alive. I was on a morphine drip and the trips it delivered had me enjoying movies inside my head. Movies in garish color, movies in which I sailed and swam and flew, all at the same time. I was lying on a Striker frame, an old-fashioned stabilizing contraption the hospital personnel had dusted off and hauled up from the basement where it had long been stored.

For the most part, Striker frames had been replaced by electric circle beds in which an immobilized patient's position is changed every eight hours to help prevent blood clots forming in the limbs and the lungs. My condition was far too precarious for a circle bed. The doctors feared the movement the bed made—that is, taking me, sandwiched between two surfaces, from a prone position, to an upright one, to deposit me face down—was not gentle enough to prevent my spinal cord from being severed.

In a Striker frame, the motion was not circular, but from side-to-side, entailing a quick, deft movement circumventing the slow, inch by inch, gravity-inducing one. I lay on a metal frame topped by a mattress, a bed as narrow as a camp cot, and when the time came for a change of position, another such frame, this one with a hole at the top for my face to poke through, was placed over me and lashed down. Like a trout frying in a wire basket, that's how I was flipped over.

I stayed in the ICU for two weeks, then was transferred to a private room. The morphine dosage was diminished from IVs to hypodermics every four or six hours. Oh, how I loved and adored whomever ventured in with my deliverance! When I'd hear her or him approach, I was shamelessly ingratiating. "You know what, you're the greatest. You know what, you're the cutest. You know what, bar none, there's no greater, cuter person on this earth than you." I don't remember it, but there surely must have been lots of eye-rolling going on.

Yet, being out of my mind on morphine was the right thing to be when every bone in my body felt hoed under and mulched. Needless to say, my back, but also my feet, which although they'd been X-rayed and the films showed no breaks, certainly looked broken. It was the whiplash effect that bruised them so badly it looked as if I were wearing short black tennis socks, with those cute little pom-poms left off.

And there was the huge lump on my head, one so alarming that scans were taken of my head, which luckily revealed no damage. (On some days, however, I could have argued those results.) Every now and then I'd reach and gently poke the lump in disbelief. Yep. That was some goose-egg, all right.

In light of these injuries, the IBD took a miraculous hike. I don't remember a single time I was preoccupied with the old maladies. In the hospital (and I would be there until a few days before Halloween, almost three months), my life consisted of two preoccupations: keeping an eye out for my next pain shot or pain pill (I was in short time demoted from morphine to Percodan, still a pretty trip-ey drug), and screwing up my courage for my next Striker-frame turnover.

These twice-a-day flips absolutely terrified me. To put it mildly, I was frightened to death that I'd be dropped. That I'd be dropped and that what the accident had begun, the flipping-over would complete. When the team—there were four of them—came in to do their job, I'd start apologizing the minute they hit the door. I'm sorry, I'm so sorry I'm such a coward. I'd beg them, beg them! to be careful. From my restricted vantage point, I'd watch as they slipped the pins into the swivels at the top and bottom of the frame. I'd make them check once, twice, three times that the pins were locked in place. When they laid the top frame over me, secured it down at the sides, I'd lift my arms and wrap them around the edge of the frame and hang on for dear life. Each time, I insisted on a countdown to prepare myself: One, two, three, go! I'd clamp my eyes shut, hold my breath, each time awaiting the horrifying contact with the floor.

My God. It's no wonder I so looked forward to the good stuff. The good stuff kept the pain at bay, but it also gave my spirits a little boost, something I sorely needed. In the hospital, because I was forced into immobility, my point of view was narrowed to what I could see while lying on my back, to what I could see while on my belly, my face poking through that special opening. Straight, perfectly straight I had to lie. No leaving bed, no sitting up, no being propped on my side. Except for side-to-side movements, no lifting my head! In fact, having a pillow was verboten. I wasn't even allowed to lift my hips so that a bedpan could be slipped under. The Striker people had seen to that. For that, there was another opening right under my butt. A special bed pan was slipped *under* the bed and hooked into place, then, it was bombs away.

Let's face it, I was an egg in a frying pan, now sunny-side up, now easy-over down. In fact, I'd eat while facing down, my plate on a little table under the bed. The bed so narrow I could reach around the sides to feed myself. And because seeing the television screen was next to impossible, I frequently just listened to what was going on. Or I'd fumble around with the buttons on the nurse's call remote and find the radio switch and listen to that, the little amplifier right up next to my ear. I used to listen to the radio into the wee hours of the night. The Christian station was my favorite. All those songs about letting Jesus take charge of things.

A few years ago, overcome by nostalgia that had me yearning to return to places where I'd spent significant time, the hospital came to mind. On a whim, I drove over and took the elevator up to my former floor. It was an eerie visit. The hospital was undergoing renovations, and that particular wing was empty. I wandered down the long hall, past the vacant nurses' station, into the room that had been my little world. The room was smaller than I'd remembered it, a common thing when we look back. But there was the same black speckled linoleum I spent hours staring at. I gazed up at the ceiling and, sure enough, there was that same soundproofing treatment that had turned the spot above where my bed had been into what I'd decided was a camel with three humps.

Bleak as the experience was, I had had good times in the hospital. The room smelled always of flowers. Helium balloons, some with smiley faces, bobbed against the ceiling when the air fan went on. My parents were then living in Saint Louis, and Mami flew in for a week. This despite my protests that she stay away. I look back, now that my parents are gone, and think of how hard this request must have been for Mami. But the truth is, I had wanted my parents only as near as their voices over the telephone. I had not wanted them at my side, to view my broken body, to learn how shattered my married life had become.

My sister Anita lived in El Salvador and could not leave the country because of the political turmoil there, so instead of making a trip north, she used the money she would have spent on airfare to call me every day. I looked forward to her voice and our chats meant the world to me, but again, despite our closeness, I never mentioned my condition leading up to the accident, nor the fact that my husband had been ready to leave me.

Friends dropped by the hospital, and some brought books and read to me; most simply sat and brought me up to date on what was happening out there in the world. My husband came once or twice a week, and after they returned from their stay in Missouri, he'd bring the boys. They stood next to my bed, perplexed and not knowing what to say. School started soon after, and it was a good thing that their activities made it difficult to visit. No matter. We took to talking on the phone. Phone visits were better visits for my children. On the phone, my voice perky and optimistic, you'd never know how hurt I'd been.

Jim Kondrick came often, too. First, because there was the matter of the overdue translation. Then, because life's problems were throwing us more and more together.

But to be honest, he visited because we were falling in love. It had happened as we worked, as we lunched, as we sometimes had drinks after work. Slowly during these times, we opened up and spilled out to each other the contents of our hearts. So I looked forward to Jim bending over my hospital bed. And soon, the nurses, perhaps sensing that something was happening between us, took to teasing me about him. They'd help me get ready for his visits by brushing my hair and helping me don a fresh scarf. (Because washing my hair was out of the question, I wrapped my head in colorful scarves.) Or they'd hold the hand mirror up while I powdered my face and applied a little eyeliner, a few strokes of blush, some lipstick.

Even in my terrible condition, with Jim, I felt pretty and interesting and whole. All the things I'd missed about myself for so long. Each time he left, one of Wilson Learning's seminar adages came readily to my mind: "I like me best when I'm with you."

Throughout the day, the nurses would stream in, for my room had become their haven. They'd use it for sneaking a quick smoke, for sitting for a moment with their feet up, for catching a few scenes of their favorite soap. Most of all, they'd come in and tell me things. Tell me stories about their lives. About boyfriends and lovers. About kids, about husbands. Lots of times, tales of cheating husbands. Lots of times, about divorce. About the numbing loneliness that most times follows it.

While they unburdened themselves, I'd listen, my own story banging around in my heart like a caged bird bent on breaking out. I, too, was wild to take flight, to flee from a marriage in which only one person seemed to matter. With him, it was always me, me, me. With him, you, you, you became an accusation. Or so it seemed to me. Lying pinned to the cot, I plotted my escape, though the plotting terrified me. Where would I go? What would I do? How could I do it? To further add to my worries, I was soon to be encased in a body cast which I'd be wearing for four months. Trapped inside a body cast, how could I do anything at all?

And my boys. Given my condition, how could I take care of them? Dear Lord, I asked, What will happen to my boys?

• • •

I left the hospital two days before Halloween, one day before my son Christopher's thirteenth birthday. I think we had a party, but I'm not sure of it. I know we had a cake because I remember seeing a photo of me plunked ramrod in a wooden chair with a tall, straight back. In the foreground, Chris blows out his candles. While he made his wish, I surely was making mine. Help me, Jesus, help me cope with this body cast. Help me cope with this life.

The cast covered me shoulders to hips. In the front, there was an opening for my breasts. The cast had been molded over my torso while in a hyperextended position; that is, my shoulders thrown back, the small of my back pushed forward. The cast arched high off my shoulders so that I looked like a dwarf linebacker. From the look of my outwardly thrust chest, a rushing linebacker at that.

Oh, that I were as fierce and fearless as one.

Living in a body cast made mundane things difficult. Because the plaster could not be wet, because in it, I could not bend at the waist, nor reach past my fingertips, personal hygiene was the most difficult of all. Shampoos were infrequent given that to have one I had to lie on the entire length of the kitchen counter, my head hanging down into the sink. One thing about my husband, he was kind enough to shampoo my hair on a couple of occasions. The boys also pitched in sometimes, and the three of us would giggle as they lathered me up. Showers, of course, were not possible, so I'd do what I could standing in the tub, kneeling down to reach the little water I'd let run into it. And wiping after toilet use, well, let me just say that there are special contraptions made especially for this sort of complication. You get them when you make that necessary visit to the occupational therapist. Extenders, they're called. I had one for toilet use, another for pulling up my thick socks, a must in Minnesota when frigid drafts reach in to cool the floors.

Still, despite the difficulties, I went out and got myself a full-time job at Wilson Learning Corporation. Jim helped me do it by singing my praises to the boss of the international division who lived in Montreal. In hiring me, the personnel in the division swelled from two to three. I became the liaison between the home office and abroad. This position necessitated that I make frequent trips to Canada and Mexico and Central America. Which I did. In my full body cast.

I remember one trip I made and how when I left the airplane the stewardess (they were called this back then) said to me in amazement, "You're in a body cast, aren't you?" When I nodded, she said, "You poor thing."

But I didn't feel like any such thing. Even encased in plaster, I felt free and alive. Like maybe with a little help I could do anything. Though I must confess that the little help I was receiving came when I got home and the sun started to set and the bar was thrown open and out marched the gin bottle, the vermouth, the jar of plump olives. To complement the aid, there were the little pills I'd shake periodically into my palm. Prescribed pills, I must say, but pills nonetheless. Pills for pain, for sleeplessness. Darvon and Valium come to mind. Also a little wonder called Prodolina, which I'd buy, along with the D and the V, over the counter when I made business trips to Mexico. I can't believe I did this, but in Mexico I'd stock up on the good stuff, bring a suitcase stuffed with drugs back across the border, holding my breath against an inspector asking me to open up. Not one ever did. And I still can't say if that was a lucky thing or not.

Throughout all this, maybe because of it, my gut was, for the most part, quiescent, a blessing, for I can't imagine adding to my armamentarium of alcohol and drugs, the medication needed to combat an IBD flare-up.

I remember once that a woman came to Wilson Learning to give a talk on nutrition. The company was in the midst of developing a wellness seminar and a number of us had left our offices and walked over to the big conference room to hear her. The woman was expounding on the virtues of eating the right foods, on eating the correct amounts of the right foods. "In fact," she said, "thanks to my getting honest about my diet, I'm not wearing a bag." She paused for effect, then added, "I don't mean a handbag. I mean a bag hanging from my stomach."

She went on to tell the story of having ulcerative colitis, of coming to the brink of having surgery ("awful surgery" she called it), surgery that would have made her a cripple having to live with a bag. (Cripple. That's how we talked back then.)

Sitting there in the audience, I was stunned. Julie, my unseen roommate from my hemorrhoidectomy days, leaped to mind. Julie had a bag that wasn't a handbag. Was Julie now a cripple? I decided to pay very close attention to the nutritionist. I decided I very much needed to watch what I ate and how much of it I ate lest I, too, end up a cripple.

• • •

My husband and I. When all was said and done, we got a divorce, though the first step we took was to separate. For the second time. The first time had occurred two years before, when we still lived in Saint Louis. Though it was not I who'd strayed then, it was he who had insisted on that separation. Not that it appeared to trouble him, being found out. How could he *not* stray, he reasoned, given I was a mess, given I was so hard to live with, given I was . . . well, frigid. There. He might as well just come right out with it.

I remember sitting there, on our canary-yellow love seat, taking all this in. Mea culpa, mea culpa, mea maxima culpa. To further castigate myself, I might have even dashed a fist against my heart. It's all my fault. Everything's my fault.

My fault or not, I had made the best of that first separation. If a separation was a must, then I'd take mine in northeastern Missouri, in Kirksville, at my alma mater, where I'd return to get a Master's degree. I think my husband could not have cared less where I was off to, though I think he was secretly amazed that in the span of a week, I'd made a trip to the campus, leased an apartment, enrolled myself in school and found a paid teaching assistantship to boot. This extra bonus meant that my tuition would be covered as would the cost of the apartment and my living expenses. Hooray for me. I could do this on my own.

Pretty darn good the way I could function, function well, I'd venture to say, when all around me my life looked like a train wreck. But I persevered, took a full load each quarter, taught two composition classes (oh, those student essays!), took care of my boys when they moved in after school was out. In the end, I'm proud to say, I earned my degree in one year. That I graduated *summa cum laude* was frosting on my cake.

So now it was February 1977, a month away from my thirty-sixth birthday. I was faced with a second separation, this one, at my prompting. This one, the permanent one. Permanent, because, sin or not, Jim and I had now broken our marriage vows. Jim and I were now making plans to be together. Together forever. That's what we said.

I can't remember what I told the kids. What their father said. Maybe I should confess that I don't want to remember what we told the kids. Maybe something about Mom needing a break. Something about Mom finding an apartment close to work, close to the airport because she had to go on trips. The fact is that I moved out. The fact is that I moved out and left my kids with him.

It's been decades since that terrible day. And in that time I've gone over, maybe a million times, all of the scenarios about why I allowed Chris and Jon to stay behind: the house we lived in was leased, and one I could not afford to keep, my boys wished to remain in their neighborhood, have the same friends, stay put in their school. In my defense, I could add that I was still recovering from the fall, that major surgery still loomed (all that had gone before—the three-month hospital stay, the Striker frame, the body cast—all those were simply stabilization measures, my shattered spine still demanded to be fixed), that I was quite literally in pain constantly, that I was by now hooked on booze and on the pills that gave me some relief, that, in spite of the pills, in spite of my troubles, I still had to make a living. That to make a living I was frequently on a plane, while, on the other hand, my sons' father conveniently worked from home.

All compelling reasons perhaps, but reasons that don't color the fact that when my sons were thirteen and eleven I went away from them. Though I saw them often, though they came to my apartment on weekends, the fact is I never lived with them again.

History repeating itself, but in a different form.

I was fourteen when sent away. Fourteen and feeling motherless.

• • •

I moved into a studio apartment. I'd signed a lease for a year. One big room, a small kitchen, the bathroom. I furnished the place sparsely; it was all I could do. The canary-yellow love seat. A wooden coffee table. The brick-red rocker I'd lullabied my babies in. A farm table and chairs. An old breakfront. All these from my redecorating days. I bought two new items for my apartment. A single bed and a television set. Standing, quite alone, in the middle of this reality, I felt utterly lost. What had I done? Away from here, out on Lake Minnetonka, my children were perhaps stepping across the floor of their room; down France Avenue, in Edina, Jim maybe sat in his living room, having a smoke, staring off into space. His wife out in the kitchen, oblivious or not. Over in Florida and way down south in El Salvador, my parents, my sister and her family, were horrified. They could not understand what I had done, which was no wonder, given I had not once come clean and confessed the true nature of my situation. My parents wrote letters to tell me how appalled they were. Anita wrote letters to my parents saying that surely her sister had lost her mind. Mi hermana se loquió, is what she wrote.

I think my sister was not wrong. Her sister *had* gone nuts.

Her sister was as wanton as la Ziguanaba, the wailing woman in nana's old story. Like the Ziguanaba, her sister had abandoned her sons, and God's punishment was surely upon her. Is it any wonder, then, that my gut flared up once more? Back to the doctor, back on the Azulfidine, back on the Cortenemas. Up the dose, too, on the good stuff. This my own prescriptive remedy. The cocktails and wine, of course, but also the Darvon every four hours for the terrible pain. A Valium or two for anxiety. At bedtime, another for sleeping, this one washed down with my special elimination cocktail: orange juice and mineral oil. Every morning, up at five to sit on the pot for an hour or so.

I traveled a lot during that year I lived in the apartment. Canada. Mexico. Central America. Brazil even. I traveled with mineral oil and enemas and happy pills and sleepy pills. I looked forward to evenings, when work was done, and dinner meant a few cocktails to enjoy. All the while the divorce was going through. All the while my sons' hearts were breaking. Jon turned sadly silent. Christopher turned angrily vocal. He accused, "You promised, Mom. You promised me."

Promised him what?

That I'd be his mother.

• • •

August 11, 1977. A weekday afternoon and the phone jangled in my apartment. It was my parents, now living in Florida. My brother-in-law, Dr. Carlos Emilio Alvarez, had been kidnapped by guerrilla forces in El Salvador. I'm pretty sure my heart stopped at the news. In El Salvador the prelude to war had been in full swing for a couple of years. Already, three of my old schoolmates had been kidnapped and murdered. This despite all demands met and large ransoms paid. "War tax" it was called. One friend was tortured and his body dumped on the road. The second dragged out of the shower and taken away. The third buried in the back patio of the house where his captors had taken him. It would be months before the family learned his fate, or where his remains rested. Now came this news. Was it Carlos Emilio's turn?

I jumped on a plane and joined up with my parents in New Orleans, where we flew on to San Salvador and went directly to my sister's house. When we arrived, we walked through a gauntlet of security before we were allowed to reach the front door. We walked into a pall of grief and breath-stopping fear. My sister, her eyes red and swollen, a photograph of her beloved clutched to her heart, fell into our arms. Her four children—ages four to twelve—knotted around her, their eyes dull and wet and seeking answers.

We settled in to wait. Carlos Emilio's father's study had become the command post. His father, the patriarch of the Alvarez family, a coffee-growing and coffee-processing family, was the commander-in-chief.

I remember most vividly two events from that time. Me, out under the trees in the garden late at night, a transistor radio in my hands, fine-tuning to Radio Havana, straining to hear any news carrying Carlos Emilio's name. Radio Havana, we thought, might give us added information. Of course, we ran the risk of learning via this medium that the "war prisoner" had been eliminated.

A more wrenching memory is that of my sister and me in her bedroom. Drapes pulled, air still and cool. Ani and I, lying on the wide spread of her marriage bed, holding each other, Carlos Emilio's photograph between us. We whispered things. She murmured, "What will I do without him? What will I do if he's not returned?"

In the end, it was a miracle. Carlos Emilio was returned after ten days of captivity. As a condition of his release, the family paid a large ransom and a manifesto was printed in all the newspapers. When he walked shakily through the door, my sister, the children, my parents and I, we all fell on our knees as if in church. My sister called out, "Gracias, Jesús mío. En éste hogar ya brilla el sol." Thank you, my Jesus. Upon this household, the sun shines again.

The family would leave the morning after for the United States, where they would stay for a few months before returning to El Salvador.

But their peace did not last long. Three years later, in 1980, they were threatened again and this time they fled for their lives in the night, over rooftops and across properties, before a private plane whisked them out of the country. To practice medicine in the United States, my brother-in-law had to repeat his internship and residency. To comply, the family lived in Washington, D.C., and then in Columbus, Ohio. In 1986, they finally settled in Miami, where Carlos Emilio at long last was able to open his private medical practice.

• • •

Back in Minnesota, it seemed the sun would never shine in my world, though in the fall there was a glimmer when Jim left home and moved into his own apartment. Six months later, he resigned from Wilson Learning and set up his own translation and consulting business. A few months after that, when my lease came up for renewal, I moved in with him.

Jim and I. Starting on our way to forever.

• • •

The surgery for my back finally came to pass six months after we moved in together. Seven hours of sawing, chiseling, carving and cleaning up called *laminectomy, facetectomy,* and *hemi-laminectomy.* The result was a spinal decompression. But before opening me up, my surgeon insisted I get clean of my drug addiction, which I did. Boom. Cold turkey. For about a week, I flopped and jerked around like something electrified before my system realized that, hey, this gal means business. No more Darvon. No more Valium. No more Prodolina. Jim was proud of me. I was proud of myself.

The surgery made all the difference. After I healed, the pain disappeared. Not so the pain in my heart at the separation from my children. For that pain, there was the bar in the living room and the bottles in the bar. Jim was a hearty drinker, so after work each day, the two-person party would commence. After half a drink, as the saying goes, I was feeling no pain. Had an armed bandit made his way into our house, I would have jumped up on a countertop and wagged a finger at him.

In the meantime, two legal actions were underway: Jim's divorce was in the works, as was the suit I'd brought against the person who'd built the deck from which Eddie and I fell. It appears the railing of the deck had been ill-constructed. The crossbeams had not been screwed to the uprights as was code-compliant, but simply nailed, and *from the outside in.* Over time, the weight of people leaning against the railing had caused it to slowly pull loose. It was Eddie's and my misfortune to provide the last straw that broke, not the camel's back, but my own.

When the settlement came in and, almost concurrently, Jim's divorce, Jim and I bought a condominium (where we still live). We married on May 25, 1980, at the home of dear friends. The day was glorious as we stood under a spread of giant cottonwoods, their white seedlings fluttering down on us as if in benediction. In attendance were my parents and our children. My two, and Jim's three, his a few years older than mine. None of the seven were necessarily thrilled at the event, but they were there, and at times I saw smiles on their faces. Given the circumstances, I couldn't ask for more.

• • •

My tilting world began to straighten itself out once we moved into the condo. We had used all the settlement money for a down payment and somehow this very painfully gained nest egg provided a strange sense of accomplishment: I had literally broken my back for a home of my own. How many can make a claim like that? Who would *want* to make a claim like that?

One of the reasons we had chosen the condo was that I was only minutes away from Wilson Learning, plus the grounds were beautiful, as was the grand recreation center. Unlike any condo in the Twin Cities, Edina West has an outdoor *plus* an indoor tennis court and swimming pool. There are saunas, his, hers, co-ed, a handball court, a whirlpool, his and her exercise rooms with all manner of equipment. And to connect the four buildings to the center, we have underground tunnels, which are just the ticket when temperatures hover at zero or below. A common occurrence, of course, in Minnesota.

I was happy to have this kind of place to lure my sons over. Though our apartment did not have an extra bedroom, we bought a sleeper sofa for the den. Not that they used it often. They were still in Mound, living now with their father and his new wife. At seventeen and fifteen, it was not their parents' company that Chris and Jon sought; it was their school chums and their school activities. Football, wrestling, drama, band. When I was not traveling, Jim and I were frequent spectators at these events.

Odd as this might be, on a couple of occasions, when the ex and his wife took a trip, it was I who would pack a bag and drive out for sleepovers with my sons. I'd make dinner. We'd watch TV. We'd be together. Sometimes, it would strike me how out-of-whack this scenario was. I'd be lying on the couch, after the kids were asleep, and I'd look around the room, spotting in the gloom some of my left-behind possessions: that lamp, that chair, this coffee table, that side table. Items that I'd bought and renovated myself. *What's wrong with this picture?* I'd ask myself. But then I'd go on to say to myself, *I don't want to think about that,* and I'd drop the subject, just like that. Too painful. Too stressful. A subject too close for comfort.

I remember one time I was out there. I was doing the dishes after dinner. I'd washed them and dried them and was putting things away. I opened the cutlery drawer and found, way back beyond the daily-used items, twelve silver demitasse spoons I'd received for my wedding to the boys' father. The spoons were held together by a rubber band. Each had a little coffee bean at the top of the handle. The spoons had come from El Salvador, sent to me by Salvadoran friends.

Finding them caused a burst of anger to fill up my chest, and so I picked them up and stuffed them into my purse. Those spoons belonged to me. I was taking those spoons back.

Why, then, the spoons and not my sons?

It was this question, which directly or indirectly I sometimes asked of myself, that made me look forward so much to the end of the day, to the opening of the bar. Now that the happy pills were a thing of the past, there was always the booze for denial maintenance.

• • •

After moving into the condo, I started writing fiction again, that old murder mystery set in Missouri that I'd stashed away. Late at night, or in between the trips my job required, I'd tap, tap, tap the story out. I owned an IBM Selectric, but Jim took pity on me one day and bought me a computer, a huge apparatus called a Vector. To complement it, he bought a clunky printer, the kind that used the sheets of paper that fold into an interminable fan. When the thing was printing out, you could hear it in all corners of the apartment. But no matter. I was in heaven writing my novel. I'd gone back to my writing group and they, and Jim, who was my first reader, were so encouraging that Jim made me an offer I could not refuse: "Quit your job at Wilson Learning, and I'll support you until you get published."

Sweeter, more helpful words could not have fallen on these ears. I took Jim up on his offer and started writing full-time. It was a good thing to be working at home. Over the years, managing ulcerative colitis and a job at the same time was becoming more and more difficult. There was the cramping and bloating and nausea, and how can you be pleasant and cheerful, how can you be effective with clients, when your mind is awhirl with the need to use the bathroom? With the fear that you might not make it to the bathroom in time?

That very thing had happened to me in the Cayman Islands. Jim and I were there with the owner of the company, Jim consulting, and me just doing my job. We had all been out to dinner, a relaxing time with good food, tall drinks, the night silky against our arms, the ocean rhythmically providing an aural backdrop. Dinner over, we were walking to the car, when the urge assailed me so strongly that I lurched back to the women's room, but this time, I didn't even make it to the door.

That night I learned how to clean up in a bathroom stall. How to be thankful for a long silk scarf. How a scarf and (I'm sorry to have to admit this) the very water in the toilet can be of service. How it's not such a bad thing to discreetly toss nice panties and a beautiful scarf into a wastebasket.

That's the kind of unpleasantness I'd been living with, so, needless to say, staying home to write, my own bathroom only steps away from the Vector, was a little slice of heaven.

We had two full bathrooms in the condo; I set mine up for extended sitting-on-the-throne sessions. We had a cat by then, a Lynx-point Siamese named Pancho Villa, and he didn't mind the time he spent on the big fluffy rug. I brought in a two-shelf bookcase and stocked it with my favorite tomes of poetry. With crossword puzzles and magazines and a notebook and pens. I indulged in a padded toilet seat: easy on the tush and, in the winter, oh, so much warmer than the regular kind. The previous condo owner had installed a phone jack in the bathroom, so I bought a lime-green Princess phone (you have to be royalty to sit on a throne) and voilà! I had it all: my kitty's company, my big mug of strong coffee, the puzzle, the newspaper, the phone for chatting away.

And, of course, the stacks of rolls of Charmin (the quilted kind), boxes of Kleenex, the cylinders of Tucks.

I tell you, if organization and being prepared is your game, then this is what you do when a disease puts bathroom-use at the top of your daily priority list.

• • •

About this time, I found Dr. Robert Mackie. My symptoms were worsening and the doctor I'd been seeing—a colon and rectal surgeon, actually—recommended I switch over to a gastroenterologist. I took to Bob Mackie right away. He's a Gary Cooper kind of guy: tall, slim, with an open, yet controlled demeanor. The perfect complement to my own ebullient self, which can sometimes turn rambunctious. On that first visit, Mackie did a quick flexible sigmoidoscopy, a much easier test than the old kind performed with a rigid instrument. The "flex-sig" scope is bendable and thus conforms itself to the convolutions of the colon, a much less painful journey. And no more butt-up-in-the-air position. Now, I laid on my side, tastefully draped. The test took only a few minutes, given it was the sigmoid portion of the colon he was checking. For the uninformed, the sigmoid (from the Greek letter *sigma*) is the S-shaped section of the colon between the descending section and the rectum. We're talking ten or so centimeters, here.

What Mackie encountered that day when he scoped me was a very active case of rectal ulcerative colitis. That was the good news: that it appeared as though the disease was restricted to the sigmoid section of the colon. To confirm this, he scheduled a colonoscopy for a week later.

A colonoscopy is a more invasive test in which the scope (with a tiny camera on the end) travels along the entire colon and the image of its passing appears on a monitor. Think of a car, a compact, traveling through a tunnel. A very twisty, and in my case, because of disease, a lumpy-walled tunnel.

Way back then, in the early eighties, having a colonoscopy was a royal pain in the butt. First, and really foremost, there was the question of colon preparation, for it was imperative, then as now, that the intestinal track be completely clean. To accomplish this, you had to drink, in a very short period of time, what amounted to an ocean. *Go Lightly* it was called, and it came in a gallon jug that grew salty, saltier and saltiest with each eight-ounce drink. You do the math. There are 128 ounces in a gallon. I think I managed to keep most of that down. I think the dosing took about three hours. Soon after that, it was throne-time, and allow me to tell you that "going lightly" does not remotely get it said.

The procedure itself was not a walk in the park, but it was made bearable by the Valium administered directly into a vein. Oooo, mama. The good stuff again.

Almost twenty years later, the procedure has changed radically. The colon-cleansing drink is now down to eight ounces. And those are palatable ounces due to some kind of flavoring. The scope itself has undergone changes as well, changes making it easier for both physician and patient to manage. The Valium, well, the Valium is what it is, and doctors are good about giving the patient a dose that allows for a very pleasant trip.

So, if you need a colonoscopy (in fact, if you're over forty you *should* undergo one) as a colon-cancer prevention measure, don't worry. Be happy.

In the end, the test verified what Bob Mackie had surmised when he did the flex-sig: the disease was restricted to the rectum.

Enter my long acquaintance with prednisone, a synthetic hormone commonly called a "steroid," and very similar to cortisone, the hormone that the body manufactures. Both ulcerative colitis and Crohn's disease are autoimmune diseases (rheumatoid arthritis, chronic fatigue syndrome, lupus, fibromyalgia, multiple sclerosis, myasthenia graves, psoriasis, to name a few, are as well), and prednisone suppresses the production of antibodies that might cause the disease. (What a difference in thinking from the old belief that IBD was caused by personality quirks.) Taking prednisone, a high daily dose to get things rolling, dramatically reduced the inflammation in my rectum. That translated into less pain and less rectal bleeding. A minor miracle.

But prednisone is a double-edged sword. On the one hand it was a miracle in what it could do *for* me, but it was also a nightmare in what it could do *to* me. What I'm talking about are those dreaded side-effects.

• • •

Sharking. That's what I called it when all the prednisone had kicked in, the 80 milligrams of it, and I was on the prowl, unable to settle down, like sharks on the move, since sharks never sleep. Once, heavy into sharking, I pushed a cart into Byerly's, one of Minneapolis's upscale grocery stores. Ravenous, I rushed straight to the deli section and into the cart went a wedge of Gorgonzola, a square of Dublin white-cheddar, a small tub of green olives stuffed with garlic, another of sun-dried tomato spread, a little tray of sushi; the California rolls looked nice. The crackers too, the ones sprinkled with cracked pepper. On to the takeout desserts, where I plucked up the flourless chocolate cake with the ganache frosting. Speeding past the meat and fish counters, as selections there necessitated cooking, I made it to the fruit, where berries glistened under their plastic wraps: plump blackberries, strawberries big as preemie fists, blueberries about to burst. I yanked three plastic bags from the roll and filled them so full, I had trouble with the twisty ties. The dairy case beckoned. There, I picked up a cute little glass bottle of Devon cream for the berries, whole milk to go with the cake, and, what the hell, the chocolate milk as well. Nearing the frozen foods, I turned the cart so quickly I slammed the corner of it into the side of the ice-cream case. A jarring jolt, for sure, but that did not deter me from Ben and Jerry's Rocky Road, from the quart with my name on it. Mission accomplished, I paid up and headed to the car and unlocked the door. The overhead light came on to help me see as I stashed my loot.

I glanced at the clock. It was almost 3 a.m.

When I got home, Jim was slumped on the couch in rumpled pajamas. He looked puzzled and bereft. "I woke up and you weren't there. I looked all over for you. I was just now deciding what to do."

I plopped down next to him and propped my head against his comforting bulk. "I'm sorry. I couldn't sleep again and I was hungry."

"Where did you go?"

"To Byerly's."

"God, Sandy."

"I know."

"What did you get?"

"Lots of goodies." It was the prednisone that made me do it; the prednisone that caused me to eat goodies that were not good for my gut, nor good for my weight. I had put on fifteen pounds. That's a lot of pounds when you're only five feet tall. My face was a full moon. There was a hump rising across my shoulders. The tops of my arms, well, they didn't even look like my arms. To tell you the truth, I was pretty disgusted with myself. But still, I couldn't stop myself from overeating. And I couldn't stop the sharking. All day long, round and round I'd go. At night, I was up, down. Then up until the sun rose. By that time, oh, what the hell, I just stayed up.

Sitting on the couch at 3:30 a.m., Jim laid a warm arm around my shoulders. "I'll unload the groceries," he said. "If I know you, there's probably ice cream in there." He gave my knee a pat and rose from the couch.

"You got that right," I said.

• • •

In addition to the prednisone, Bob Mackie switched me from Azulfidine to 6-mercaptopurine, or 6-MP. That drug had less gastric side-effects than the Azulfidine, but it did lower my blood counts, which was not a good thing. To keep a check on the levels, I had to visit my general practitioner's office. There I popped in once a week and headed directly to the lab where the technician dug around in my arm. Remembrance of Harry past. From the get-go my veins were slippery, much as Harry had learned, but these frequent tests made matters much worse. Now, before setting off for the lab, I'd warm up a hot-pack and place it on my arm (the right arm, the one with the best sites) to bring the veins up to the surface. And I'd insist on a butterfly needle, the thin, thin kind used on babies and frequently on people undergoing extensive chemotherapy. Usually those two ingredients made for best results. But, I tell you, those visits got awfully old, me squirming around on the seat as the vampire tried to get her fill. On those days, the phrase, "I got it!" was music to my ears.

As my blood levels dropped, so did my stamina. It drained huge amounts of energy to get up out of bed. To put in throne-time, to take a shower, to dress. To turn things around, Bob Mackie ordered weekly iron injections, same as the Puerto Rican doctor had prescribed when I was nine. Just like those, these painful shots turned my buttocks as dark as molasses again. This time, I had to go it alone, for there was no Abuelita to hold me down and help me wail away. But the iron helped, and so I was able to get up each day, go through my morning ritual, before showing up for work, work that took me into the den, to my desk with the Vector and the in-basket with all my novel's pages piling up in the tray.

When I completed the book, I wrote for an application to Bread Loaf Writer's Conference in Vermont. It was a naive, yet cheeky thing to do, for Bread Loaf was then the premiere workshop destination for any writer. Get into Bread Loaf, it was then thought, and you might be on your way to fame and fortune. Founded in 1926, its faculty has included Robert Frost, Archibald MacLeish, Norman Mailer, Shirley Jackson and John Gardner, among other luminaries. For two weeks in August, the conference takes place on the summer-campus of Middlebury College with its rolling verdant lawns, yellow clapboard cottages named Cherry, Birch, Maple and Larch, all front-porched and as charming as small inns. An idyllic, New England campus with the Green Mountains lumbering on the horizon, all misty and mystic-looking in the early mornings.

Late in 1982, I sent in my application along with the first 30 pages of the novel. That following spring, I learned I'd made it in. The news was stunning. The faculty that summer would include Tim O'Brien, John Irving, Linda Pastan, Robert Stone, Nancy Willard and Wilma Holitzer, to name a few. It was both exhilarating and terrifying to think I'd be attending workshops by these writers who, as far as I was concerned, were as famous as rock stars. Most terrifying of all was that my manuscript would be critiqued. By whom, the admittance letter did not say.

Once on campus, I was dumbstruck by the literati I'd come upon in the dining room (writers actually eat!), in the recreational barn, on the walks to and from my room. Each time I sat in the barn, listening in awe to one of the famous writers reading behind the podium, I'd imagine myself alone with him, with her, my manuscript like an offering between us.

Five days after my arrival, I found out that it would not be one of the top faculty who would discuss my book with me. When the time came, I found myself sitting in one of the quaint rooms at Tamarack, the big house on the hill. I found myself facing one of the staff associates, an author I'd never heard of before coming to Bread Loaf. An author I've never heard of since.

The critique session turned out to be a nightmare. The man called my work "shit." His very word. He went on to tell me, for a full two hours, how flushable my novel was. I sat before him, numb with shock. As if to console me, the sun streamed through a window and deposited a golden square at my feet. I listened to him go on and on. "See this scene here? This is ridiculous. This would never happen." As he droned on, I bit my lower lip, trying to keep from weeping. I set my face in a mask, a dumb smile plastered on it, a smile that was meant to please him, to show him what a big girl I was. A big girl capable of taking this devastating news.

When the ordeal was over, and we were both standing on the lush lawn that swept all the way down to the main inn, he topped my torture by saying, "I hope I haven't been too easy on you." Then off he went, merrily it seemed to me, down the hill to Treman, the cottage that was off-limits to us common folk, for it was the watering hole for the powers that be.

Recently, in an old file folder, I found some yellowed papers on which I'd written my account of that afternoon. I titled it, "This is how it happened." I began, "I'm ready for my critique session. I've been working on this novel for three years. I'm on re-write eleven. How I pray for good news."

When I returned home, my gut in turmoil from another flare-up, I decided to stop writing, thinking, how can I be a writer if I write "shit"? But Jim said, no, you can't do that. My writing group wouldn't hear of it. Chris and Jon were away at college. Chris in Colorado Springs, Jon in Boston, but even over the phone both of them said, "Mom, you can't give up."

I took two weeks off from writing, staying mostly in bed. I was back on the Cortenemas so I had an excuse to lay quiet and still. Plenty of time to mull things over. To try to make sense of the writing life: Was it really for me? Did I have the tenacity, the drive, to actually be published? Was I talented enough to succeed? As I pondered these questions, one thing became clear to me: the man had been right, although he could have delivered the news in a gentler, kinder fashion. The truth was my novel was not publishable; the writing was not distinguished and the story was not a memorable one. I could certainly do better.

Lying in bed, I thought back to El Salvador, and the servant's oak table, their stories rising up in my mind like photographs. I thought of those dear, tender women.

I realized that I'd held their stories deep in my heart. It was from this place that I'd write, I determined. No more meaningless murder story set in Missouri. Instead, I'd turn to my own true stories, my Latino stories. And to do it, I'd take Benítez, my mother's maiden name. In this way, I'd claim my own Latino heritage. Empowered by this decision, I finally got out of bed.

I decided to give my failed manuscript a proper burial. I went out and bought a good storage box. I lit a candle and placed all those pages into the box. I said a prayer, thanking my book, thanking it for teaching me to keep faith with the page, for showing me that the way to write a novel is to sit down and write it. I placed the box under my bed. I still sleep over it to this day.

Feeling strengthened and hopeful, I began to write *A Place Where the Sea Remembers.* A novel with Remedios, the healer, at its heart. Remedios, so like my old nana, the laundress. Nana who allowed me my thumb in my mouth. Nana who, like Remedios, believed it was stories that can save us.

• • •

In the hospital, perhaps my surgery was finally coming to its conclusion. Perhaps Dr. Madoff was heading from the surgery field to peel off his gloves. Perhaps the anesthetist was extracting the breathing tube from my wind pipe, the circulating nurse and the scrub tech were busily tallying instruments, basins, drapes towels, sponges and pads. Perhaps the stark, shadowless light above the surgery table was dimmed and I went swirling into the memory of that day when I had traveled to Maryland to visit, for the first time, my twin sister's grave.

THE GRAVE WAS HARD TO FIND. I had a map of the cemetery, with a circle around Section N, Lot 364, Site 3, and I'd walked back and forth over the indicated area, clutching my tote bag and a small bouquet of lilies of the valley, but hadn't yet come upon the round plaque set into the ground with "SUSANA BENITEZ ABLES, March 26, 1941–May 3, 1941" inscribed in top and bottom arcs upon it.

I looked out across the cemetery, where no grave stones, only ground markers, were permitted, my sight sweeping over the leafless trees. The grounds looked forlorn under the low Maryland sky. The winter's snow and ice had left their marks: bare spots and grassy areas pale and patchy. It was early April, and a few dogwoods bloomed, however. Their hopeful white flowers grew terraced along the branches and floated above them. A solitary black bird perched on a nearby branch cawed encouragement as I stepped carefully around the markers.

Here lay Mary Crittenden who died in 1947, at only forty-two years of age. There David Lamb who died in 1944. Edith Taber in '45, and Emma Fertig in '46. I imagined Susana, having been laid to rest only a few years earlier, greeting them all when their funeral processions rolled up.

Almost under my feet, lay the grave of tiny Pamela who lived for only two days in December of 1951. "Our Precious Daughter" was etched upon her plaque. I pictured a young man and woman, much like my own parents in 1941, huddled together, their heads bowed, their hearts broken. What words of comfort did Susana have for them? I wanted to think she breathed something soothing about resignation and acceptance. But all I could think of her saying is, It isn't fair.

As if he'd been watching, the groundskeeper came up and I showed him the map and asked for help. He studied the yellowed document Daddy had sadly handed me years before. Like a homing pigeon, the man went directly to the spot. He pointed down at Susana's grave. "Here you go." He stepped back, went off, giving me my privacy.

It was just as Daddy had described it. The bronze disc gone to green patina, the name, the dates, the small round opening in the center that, when I hunkered down and poked a finger through and lifted, revealed a bronze vase. I pulled it out and set it right, emptying into it the bottle of water I'd carried in my tote. I filled the vase with my store-bought lilies and their delicate sweetness perfumed the space around me. Around us.

Susana and me together, a few hand-spans of packed earth between us. Together again since the time we'd floated in the watery haven of our mother's womb, our hearts beating almost as one. Together again since mother's forced early labor had wrested us apart.

They had placed us in separate Isolettes, our only comfort the radiance from the 20-watt bulbs positioned in our incubator tops. They had wrapped us so snugly in swaddling cloths (around and around our little bodies, up and around our tiny faces) that we had looked like white panatellas. We had been so small, Daddy had said, that we could have fit into cigar boxes. Back then, our bird-bone breasts heaved with the difficulty of our breathing. Our hearts were fairy bell clappers knocking quickly in our chests.

So many years later, my heart filled with longing and regret. I had lived a life while Susana moldered there. As ever, I had felt the guilty weight of it. Why Susan and not me? Why Susana at all?

At my sister's grave, I had settled myself down over her. From my tote, I pulled a shoe box containing mementoes, photographs and letters, for I had come to share flashes and fragments of my life. Come to recount my own true stories.

• • •

In Minnesota, my stories for fodder, I started entering fiction-writing contests, the ones sponsored by various state organizations. I'm a lucky gal to live in a state that so generously supports the arts in general, and literary arts in particular. In Minnesota, we have the McKnight Foundation, the Bush Foundation, the Minnesota State Arts Board, the Jerome Foundation.

And we have the Loft Center. A place for readers and writers alike. The Loft provides writing workshops of all kinds, readings by local writers and national literati. They also sponsor a number of contests and awards. One of them, the Mentor Award, pairs emerging writers in fiction and poetry with nationally known writers who come in to do workshops with the contest winners. I began sending my writing to the Loft for this award, and on my third try, I received a call that I had won. I'm quite sure that my squeals of delight broke the eardrum of the person who made the call. I was four years into the writing, four years into Jim's financial sponsorship. Needless to say, it was a great day when I told him that someone, in this case Ron Hansen, the author of *Mariette in Ecstacy,* deemed my writing good enough for an award.

To help Jim out, I took a job with COMPAS—Poets and Writers-in-the-Schools. I needed the work, for Chris and Jon were now in college, and I was helping with the expense.

The COMPAS program provided a roster of writer biographies to the public schools, grades K-12. Teachers selected the writer they wished to work with, and off the writer would go to spend a week at the school. The work, though very satisfying, was exhausting. In my case, it meant traveling out of town. Holing up in a motel. Being at school by 7:30. Working until 4. Grabbing a quick supper, before falling into bed. A motel room bed. And the job entailed the preparation of several lesson plans given that I was visiting a number of different grades. Sometimes I went to towns housing canneries and the migrant workers who worked in them. Often the children of these workers were in my classes. Their whole faces lit up when I spoke to them in Spanish.

In spite of the joy I felt to be doing work that was so worthwhile, accomplishing it while ill and on the road was, to put it mildly, highly inconvenient. It was the prednisone, and the boost it gave me, that made all that activity possible.

In this case, sharking was a very good thing.

• • •

In 1988 my drinking had become a real problem. I was having blackouts on a regular basis. Have a drink, two drinks max, and boom, the curtain went down and though I'd still be functioning, I could not later remember anything I'd done. What I'd done, I didn't want to know about.

One day, my dear friend Judy and I were trudging over the streets of her neighborhood. It was an early May morning and we were doing some serious walking in the warm Minnesota sun. Judy maintained a brisk pace, but I was having trouble keeping up. My head pounded. My skin was so sensitive that if you touched me, I would have shivered.

The night before I had celebrated my forty-seventh birthday with a much-belated party and with plenty of champagne. Over the years, my drinking preferences had included martinis, brandy Alexanders, Manhattans, red wine (only good cabernets), white wine (only good chardonnays and icy cold at that). Now I was nuts about champagne. I couldn't afford the expensive kind, so I'd settled on the Spanish brand Freixnet.

"Wait up," I said to Judy. I was certain I could feel the grit of the pavement right through the soles of my Reeboks. Judy put on the brakes. She turned to look at me.

A wave of nausea engulfed me and I bent over and grasped my ankles. "God."

"What's wrong?"

I looked up at her. She was not smiling. "I think I'm getting the flu," I said. That morning there was an unspoken tension between us, and my mind was wild with what my mind was always wild about after I'd been drinking: What did I do? What did I say? Did anyone notice?

Judy started down the street again. We went one block, two. The trees along the sidewalk were budding. Their tender greenness assaulted my eyes. The warbling robins sitting on the branches sounded like fog horns. After minutes of silence, I asked Judy a question: "Do you think I'm getting the flu?"

"I have to say I don't." She did not look at me when she stated this.

I couldn't bear what I knew was coming, so I changed the subject. "You left my party early." There. Switch the focus to one of blame and all would be well.

"I *had* to leave early."

"Why?" I felt suddenly sorry for myself: birthday girl, abandoned.

Judy stopped and faced me. "I left because I couldn't stand to see what you were doing. I couldn't stand to hear what you were saying."

"What?"

"You were bumping into things, Sandy. You were slurring your words so bad nobody could understand you."

The blood drained from my head. From the tip of my toes, shame rose and filled me. I doubled over again. This time I was really going to be sick.

"Sweetie," she hunkered down and hugged me.

"I'm so sorry. I don't want to hurt you. I hate having to hurt you."

"It's okay."

"No, it's not okay. You're not okay. You need help. You have to get help."

I simply nodded my head against her shoulder.

"I'll do anything to help you. Anything. I'll go with you to AA. I'll even call and find a meeting we can both go to."

My shoulders heaved as I began to sob, as the pain of the undeniable truth wracked me. "Oh, God. Oh, God."

We were hunched down by the side of the road, and Judy held me tight, albeit awkwardly. After a time she extended a leg and dug into a pocket of her warm-ups and handed me a tissue. "Oh, God, Jude."

"I know, I know." She rubbed little circles over my back.

I blew my nose loudly. Presently I said, "Enough of this." I hauled myself up, pulling her up with me. I tried to smile, but it was no use.

"We'll get help, okay?" she said.

I blew my nose again, then pocketed the tissue. "I promise you one thing, Jude. I promise I'll call AA. When I get home, okay?"

"Okay."

But I didn't call AA. When I got home, I called Hazelden Treatment Center and got an appointment that very afternoon with a counselor for an "appraisal" of my situation. Before the day was over, I'd been accepted into the program. After hearing my story, the counselor said, "We don't like to put a label on people, but I think you really need us. We have an opening next week. You can start then."

That night, when Jim arrived home from work, I broke the news. He was having a martini. I was having a beer. It was the last drink I've had. And that was seventeen years ago.

• • •

Stopping drinking was good for my gut. It was very good for my life, though getting sober involved my getting real with myself.

When I was finally ready to put the glass down, when I was finally ready to try, to *try,* not to raise it back up to my lips, it was then that I began to understand who I had been and who I had become. A girl cast away long ago? A woman betrayed? Broken? Ill? To all counts, yes, but over and above it, I was a woman who had left her sons. I'd left my sons ten years before and had then myself become the betrayer, the breaker of precious bonds. It's what I had come to believe, though over the years, my sons have argued the point. Argued it, sometimes vehemently.

La Ziguanaba. Nana's old story. La Ziguanaba left her children and would roam the riverbanks in search of them. My sister was right. *La Sandy se loquió.* Much like la Ziguanaba, Sandy went mad. I had left my children, and the river I haunted was the stream that filled my glass every day after five.

I'm a novelist, and oh, that I could rewrite that plot line of my life.

When I gathered Chris and Jon and told them my plans for rehab, they both nodded, as if they'd always understood. There were tears in Chris's eyes. Jon said something for both of them that I'll take to my grave.

"Ma," he said, "when you go into treatment, you'll be getting lots of therapy. When you do, don't ever talk yourself into thinking we don't love you."

I ask you: What had I done to deserve sons like these?

• • •

So maybe it *was* redemption I obtained at Hazelden, but it was my sons' and Jim's acceptance and support that helped me see my way. I know I obtained sobriety there, that I began to forgive myself there. But these hard-won blessings were not enough to cure my illness. Alcohol or not, I was still sick. And getting sicker by the day. So sick I had to be hospitalized a few times and hooked up to the IV with the prednisone. In a day, I'd blow up like a balloon, my wiring so jacked up, I'd get out of bed and do laps while pushing the IV pole along beside me. Zip, zip down the hall, circling the nurses' station, the nurses looking up from their chart-keeping in puzzled amazement. Slap, slap went my slippers as I flew round and round until I'd exhaust myself.

Back in my room, still revved up from my furious workout, I'd call my cousin Peg Evans, who lives in Miami. She is a relaxation therapist who works with hospitals, helping patients ready themselves for tests or for surgery. Peg has a program called *Blue Wave Relaxation,* and over the phone she would guide me in visualization, her gentle lulling voice washing over me and calming me down.

During these hospital stays, Bob Mackie was, of course, my physician, and he came in daily to see how I was doing, taking the time to sit and chat. It's what I liked about him. He'd sit back in the chair as if he had no other place to go. And we would have a conversation. Not him lording his doctorship and knowledge over me, but a real conversation in which we tried together to find solutions for my worsening state. I could participate in this, because I was an informed patient. Something I think all patients should be.

It was very obvious that my options were running out. The prednisone was making a mess of me. Because of it, I had bouts of arthralgia, terrible pain in my hands and my feet as if I had rheumatoid arthritis. My mother suffered from this malady, and so we'd compare notes and, sure enough, my pain was like hers, though my joints were not inflamed and growing gnarled as hers. And my immune system was totally out of whack. At times, I'd have unexplained fevers. Pus-filled sores on my head, once a nasty one that made my nose look like Bozo the Clown's.

The 6-MP was losing its effect. My rectum was so swollen, its lining sloughing off so severely, that there was great risk the colon wall would perforate. Worse was the possibility that the whole shebang would bloom into colon cancer. The inflammation narrowed the passageway so much that it was extremely hard to have a bowel movement. No amount of mineral oil seemed to help. And mineral oil had its own kind of risks, for if taken just before bedtime (the logical time), the oil is so viscous it can easily be inhaled into the windpipe. Once in the windpipe, aspiration into the lungs can be the next thing. But the mineral oil didn't help. And all that straining caused me to bleed so severely that my blood counts dropped to dangerous levels. To make matters worse, I couldn't eat, knowing that what I put in my mouth would have to come out the other end, and the other end was so painfully sore, I preferred to keep myself empty.

And so I lost weight, my new diet consisting of broths, Saltines and Jell-O. I lost the fifteen pounds I had gained and then ten more and five more after that.

Given the direness of my condition, both Bob Mackie and my brother-in-law, Carlos Emilio, began to talk about ileostomy. And I? I surely heard what they had to say, but what they said seemed directed toward someone else. For me? An ileostomy for me?

No way, José.

• • •

Being this ill didn't keep me from working. No siree. I arranged my schedule around my morning ritual. While I'd had to drop the traveling out of town, I visited local schools to talk to students, to confer with faculty.

And I finished *A Place Where the Sea Remembers* and it was making the rounds of New York publishers. The news from them was not good. All of them had turned the book down, although with encouraging comments about the writing and the characters. The major problem seemed to be that the novel, because it is set in Mexico, and the cast of characters all Mexican, was "too foreign," and, because it was, it would get lost on their lists. "Getting lost" meaning it would not sell well.

After ten turndowns, I pulled the manuscript from circulation and gave it to my friend and fellow-novelist Mary Rockcastle, who read it and pronounced it wonderful. She then rushed it over to Coffee House Press, a small independent press in Minneapolis, and hand-delivered it to Allan Kornblum, the publisher. Mary said that Allan was always swamped with submissions; she said I might have to wait as much as a year for a response from him. I told her it didn't matter, what was one more year, when I'd already waited thirteen?

I put the book and Allan Kornblum out of my head and went about my business, business that took me a week later to Fargo, North Dakota. To the Plains Art Museum. They were running an exhibit of Latino art and thought I might complement it by giving a talk on Latino stories. Jim and I made the five-hour car trip together. He drove because my back usually gave out when I had to drive for that long a time.

The staff of the museum was gracious and welcoming. Chagrined, too, when only one soul showed up for my talk. I gave it anyway, of course. My full standard presentation, with the same enthusiasm as if the place were packed.

I was dejected on the drive home. Sick and tired, too. Sick of being sick. Tired of the mountain that my struggle with getting published had become. Thirteen years had gone by since Jim made his offer: quit your job and I'll support you until you get published. Thirteen years, two manuscripts, one forever under my bed, the other turned down time after time.

We were halfway home when I said to Jim, "You know what? I think I'm going to forget the writing. I think I'll call Wilson Learning and take them up on that job." The company had been calling, asking if I might consider facilitating workshops in Mexico.

On the road from Fargo, Jim said, "I think you're right. I think it's time to hang it up. Call Wilson Learning next week."

When we got home, the little red light on my

answering machine was blinking. I rewound the tape to find a message that changed my life.

"This is Allan Kornblum. I want to buy your novel."

As exclaimed Lewis Carroll in his poem, "Jabberwocky, "O frabjous day! Callooh! Callay!" Praised be Coffee House Press. Praised be my little book. It made quite a splash. When it was published, in the fall of 1993, the reviews were glowing. The novel won the Minnesota Book Award and the very first Barnes & Noble Discover Award. In addition, it was nominated for the Los Angeles Times First Fiction Award. This generated lots and lots of press, both local and national. It also brought me to the attention of New York agents, and because of it, I signed with Ellen Levine and that partnership has made all the difference to my career.

And Jim? I've often asked myself, had Jim known how long it would take, would he still have made his offer? I've preferred to keep that question in my head.

• • •

In October 1994 I was in Saint Louis, doing a reading for the prestigious Writer's Voice. I'd been invited to join the organization's touring group, which consisted of six writers who traveled around the country and did readings at various YMCAs.

A few days before the trip, I'd had a serious setback, so serious I could hardly make it out of bed. But hey, I wouldn't let that derail my plans. I had commitments. People were counting on me. I flew to Saint Louis the afternoon before the events scheduled for the next day. There was a newspaper interview in the morning, a radio show in the afternoon, and in the evening, the reading and reception.

When I got into town, I went immediately to the hotel and fell into bed. Around 9 p.m., I called room service and they brought up some chicken noodle soup and crackers. Half of it remained on my tray. In the morning, I ordered coffee and some cream of wheat. I got dressed and showed up for the newspaper interview, then came back to the hotel and into bed again. The radio show was a phoner, which meant I could sit in bed and do the talking. At seven, dressed again and with a smile on my face, I was standing at the podium reading from my book, talking about the writing life.

During the question-and-answer period, I had to literally hang on to the podium for fear that if I let go, I'd fall flat on my face.

The next day, when I arrived back in the Twin Cities, Jim took me directly to Bob Mackie's office. Bob took one look with the flex-sig and called the hospital to schedule my admittance. He alerted Robert Madoff, the colorectal surgeon, that I was on my way.

AFTER SURGERY

HOURS AFTER SURGERY, Jim sat at my side.

Jim Kondrick, mi hombre. My strong, faithful, formal man. With Jim's devotion and support, I had bloomed into a writer, a sober writer. With Jim beside me, cheering me on, I was slowly becoming all that I could be.

The big window in my hospital room was a black sheet of glass. In it were reflected the light of the fluorescent lamp above me and the glow of the votive candle Jim had set on the bedside table. A candle with the image of the Virgin Mary, her hands at her sides, palms up and emitting rays of hopeful light.

"What time is it, Jaimsey?"

"Almost midnight."

"Did we get it done?"

"We got it done." Jim bent over and pressed his lips to my forehead.

"I don't know if it hurts yet." The remains of the anesthetic made the words feel thick in my mouth.

"They gave you this pump." He held up a black cord with a bulb on top. "There's a button up here. You can press it when you need more medicine. The nurse said you can have it every four hours."

"Put it here." I patted the bed beside me. I wouldn't hesitate to take advantage of the apparatus every four hours whether in pain or not. I'd read somewhere that pain medication should be taken *before* discomfort arrived, not after. That way the patient remains comfortable and avoids the agony of waiting for pain to subside after taking a dose. Struggling in this way retards healing. That philosophy sounded good to me, being that when it comes to hurting, my name is Chicken Little.

Though I was well aware that I'd had a drug problem, it was not my intention to "start up" with the good stuff again. I'd take what was needed when appropriate. Having major surgery certainly qualified in this regard. Alcohol? Alcohol is a no-no. A no-no under any circumstances.

"Did you call Mami and Dad? The kids? Ani and Carlos Emilio?" My head was not totally clear, but I managed to get the list of names out.

"Yep. Your sister said she set the house on fire."

I chuckled. "Le prendí fuego a la casa." That's my sister's expression for when the occasion calls for more than one petitioning candle to be lit. She'd told me she would light one to la Virgen Milagrosa, the Miraculous Mother, one to the Sacred Heart of Jesus, one to San Rafael, the healing archangel, and one also to Saint Jude, the patron saint of the impossible. We're talking the tall votives, like the ones you sometimes see, all in a row, in wrought-iron stands in church niches. Thinking of all those candles, those flames, made me thirsty.

"Is there water? I need a little drink."

Jim brought me a glass with a bent straw in it. He held the glass while I took a few sips. "How's Mami?" I asked, after he pulled the glass back. Down in Miami, my mother was not well, to say the least. She suffered from rheumatoid arthritis and diabetes, plus she'd had a double mastectomy and a coronary bypass. This illness of mine had been an added stress for her.

"She's okay. She can't wait to talk with you. Your Dad, and Chris and Jon too."

I nodded, wishing my sons were near. Chris lived in Arizona, Jon in California. Yet even from afar, they'd been very much a part of helping me decide to have this surgery. Jon, in fact, had sent a teddy bear in a short hospital gown and with a wide bandage swathing her tummy and pulled down and around her butt. "See, Ma, even a bear can bear it," his accompanying card read. Chris called often, encouraging me at every turn. "And just think, Mom," he'd said on one occasion, "after they're through with you, no more pooping. That in itself makes the whole thing worth it."

"I'll call everyone tomorrow." My eyelids felt suddenly very heavy. I had trouble keeping them open.

"I talked with Carlos Emilio, by the way. He talked with Madoff who told him the surgery went very well. Madoff said there were no complications, no problems. In fact, he told me himself he gave you a nifty stoma. It's going to be your best friend, he said. Also, your bag's already in place."

"Good." The bag. I gingerly touched it with a tip of a finger. I could feel its plastic edge. I could hear its rustle. "Guess what, Jaimsey? I'm a bag lady now." My voice trailed off.

Jim kissed me again. "I think my bag lady needs her beauty sleep."

• • •

I awakened early, when the nurse came in to check my vital signs, and I lay there waiting for the big pain to hit. I remembered how painful the hemorrhoidectomy I'd had years before had been, and I was certain all the carving Madoff had done in that area would cause me agony. But, lo and behold, it did not.

"I can't believe it," I told the nurse. "My butt doesn't hurt. It just aches, that numb kind of ache, like when I used to sit on the concrete bleachers at my sons' football games. Are you sure Madoff didn't forget to do something back there?"

"Oh, no. You're all sewn up back there."

"I am? Are you sure?"

The nurse nodded. "You look like a Barbie doll down there."

That made me laugh, and laughing engaged my abdominals, and *that* was painful. "Wow," I said. "Let's go easy on the merriment."

The nurse looked at her watch. "You're due for your pain medication. You'll be doing quite a bit of moving around today. Like, pretty soon, you'll be getting up and using the bathroom." In preparation, she mercifully pressed the medication button.

When it was time for the trek into the bathroom, there was a rosy edge around the world, but I still felt that awful pull on every inch of my belly as I lifted myself out of bed. I took deep breaths and held onto the nurse all the way across the room. She helped me accommodate myself on the throne. "Whad'ya think? Think you'll be okay?"

"I'll be okay." I was huffing a little as I said this.

She closed the door.

I did my business, which now meant only #1, not bothering to lift my gown to take a look at my tummy and the bag, which surprised me. But given that this change was meant to last forever, I was in a stalling mode. There'd be all the time in the world to check out what was under there. I stood, holding on to the sink, and took a look in the mirror. Sick or not, there was always enough strength for a little makeup. My essentials were at hand, and so I pulled a comb through my hair. Gave it a pat. I squinted into the mirror and applied a round of eyeliner, then a bit of blush. Circled my mouth with lipstick. There. That was as good as it would get.

The nurse had been right. The morning was a busy one. Making his rounds, Rob Madoff came in to see me. He lifted my gown, poked gently around my belly, nodding in satisfaction. I never once looked down. He asked me to turn over on my side so he could check my butt. I turned slowly, hanging on to the metal side of the bed. *Ouch, eech, ouch, eech,* were the sounds that came out of me. I made the same ones when I rolled back over. "Well, what do you think?"

"I think you'll live, that's what I think. I think you'll be living a very nice life. No more pain and misery."

"The nurse said you've sewn me up back there just like a Barbie."

"She's right. I did."

"Well, I guess from this day on, no one can call me an asshole."

"Well they could, but they'd be wrong."

Bob Mackie strolled in a while later, when I was having a cup of coffee, the whole of my nourishment, so far. He settled himself in a chair. "Well, you did it. Good for you."

"Good for you and Madoff too. It took some convincing, but now that it's over, I'm holding you guys accountable. My brother-in-law too."

"How so?"

"Well, you all might've sold me a bill of goods, promising me that things would get so much better."

"We did our part; now it's up to you."

I knew what he was talking about. "It's all about attitude, isn't it?"

Bob Mackie nodded. "A great part of it is attitude."

I thought to myself how all my life it had been one attitude adjustment after another. Moving from Salvador to Missouri. Adjusting to the farm. Going to college. Being on my own. Getting married. Having babies. Divorce. Separation from my kids. Meeting Jim. Working. Breaking my back. Addiction. Everything in life, be it bitter or sweet, took some getting used to. We human beings like the status quo. Most of us, in fact, crave the status quo. Why else would the abused keep going back to their abusers? There's familiarity in the status quo, that's why. A certain safety in the familiar, even if it's nightmarishly familiar. Change is scary. Even if it's the happy change a vacation can bring about. Will the beds be comfortable? Can we eat the food? Will the water be safe? Will the airplane drop out of the sky? Who will take care of my kids if it does?

So, yes, we were talking about attitude adjustment, Mackie and I. "You know what?" I said to him. "When it comes to that cliché about taking lemons and making lemonade, I think I might have been in the lemonade business for a very long time."

"It would not surprise me."

"I'm going to miss you, Bob," I said at length. "I'm going to miss Jodi, too." Jodi was his nurse practitioner, and she and I had had countless talks on the phone. Me asking questions. Always me wanting to know about something or another. I was just like my father in this regard. Both of us, Curious Georges.

Mackie ran his hands back and forth along the arms of his chair. "Considering what you've been through, not seeing Jodi and me again is good news. Of course, you know, if anything comes up, we're only a phone call away."

"I know."

Mackie unfolded his lanky self out of the chair. "Well, off I go. A million miles before I sleep and all of that." He gave a little wave as he went through the door.

No question. I really was going to miss Bob Mackie.

Because of work, Jim was not coming in until late afternoon, so I spent the rest of the morning making phone calls. Chris and Jon were relieved and jokeful. "Are you getting shoes to match your bag?" Chris asked.

My parents wanted to crawl through the phone, they said. I relayed Chris's remark, and when they hung up, they were happy that I sounded happy.

My sister was managing the votives, and looking forward to her trip to Minneapolis. She'd come once I left the hospital. I was eager for her arrival. With Jim and my sister to help me get adjusted, all would be well.

When food service came in with lunch, the woman who brought it raised the head of the bed and helped me settle myself behind the table she rolled across me. I spread a hand gently over my bag, the stoma, the incision, afraid the edge of the table might do me harm. I still had not lifted my gown for a look-see, but this afternoon, nurse Susie was scheduled for a visit, and she would be giving me an extensive tour of the new surface of my belly.

"Don't worry," the person said. "I won't bump you." She set the tray down on the table. It held what looked like a Thanksgiving meal. There were turkey slices and gravy. Mashed potatoes, a puddle of butter. Bright green asparagus. Coffee. Milk. Pumpkin pie with a dollop of whipped cream. The rich aroma of the meal caused me to salivate. I gobbled the food down, emptied my coffee cup, drank the milk, as if I were a starving person, which I was. Ten minutes it took, and then I laid back against the pillows, thinking, that was the best meal of my life. Indeed, a thanksgiving meal.

Later that afternoon, before Susie arrived, I had my first stomal experience, as in when food has meandered its way from my mouth to the top of the stoma. As in when the food, or what has become of the food, drops into the bag.

It's a very peculiar feeling. A kind of puckering sensation in the belly at the stoma site. A scratchy feeling, too, but in a pulling sort of way. It feels as if something is inching forward, which it is: your masticated, semi-digested and digested food making its way out after nutrients have been absorbed by the small intestine. Actually, the very same thing happens in the colon, where all the liquid is extracted from our food, but that happens deep in the gut and most times, unless we have colic or something, we're not aware of it. But when it's happening so close to the surface of the skin, it produces that puckery, itchy kind of feeling.

It did that first time.

I was alone in the room, and I decided it was time to take a look. I pressed the button that raised me up in bed, then drew the sheet back and lifted my gown.

There it was. My bag. The plastic was see-through, and what I saw gave me a start: a green ball about the size of half my fist, bunched up so that the top part of the bag was expanded. I gulped and dropped the gown, pulled the sheet back over myself. Rang the nurses' station.

"Yes?"

"Quick. I need some help. Something's happening in my stomach." My voice was shaky. I remembered Julie's teary voice behind that pulled curtain back when I had the hemorrhoidectomy.

Two or so minutes later, nurse Susie strode briskly in. "Good timing, your call. I was just on my way to see you. What's happening?" Despite her brightness and sass, her face showed concern.

"Close the door."

She did, then walked over. "What's wrong?"

I lifted my gown. "Look at this." There the green ball was, but larger this time.

Susie's eyes lit up. "Look at that!"

"I am, I am. What is it?" There was more of that puckery feeling.

"Your stoma's working, that's what it is! That's fabulous!"

"What's with the green stuff?"

"Did you have lunch? What did you have for lunch?"

I listed the items.

"Asparagus! That's the asparagus!"

"What? What are you talking about?"

"The asparagus fibers. Actually, that's pretty good,

because serving you asparagus for your first meal was not a smart thing. It could have been tricky. You know, all those long strings that asparagus have?"

"Is that what that is? Asparagus strings?"

"Yeah. All rolled into a ball. I'm going to do something here, and don't be alarmed. It won't hurt a bit."

Before I could ask more or protest, Susie used the tip of her finger to push the green ball to the side. Under the see-through plastic, it rolled over into the bag.

"Oh, my God!" There was my stoma. Exposed. A little red plug. Under the plastic, it glistened wetly.

"Look at that!" Susie exclaimed. "Doctor Madoff did a great job. Your stoma's sitting right up there. And already it's doing its thing."

I lifted the tail of the bag and under it was the long track of my incision. Black plastic stitches poked up at intervals. The incision looked angry and mean. I lowered my gown. Laid my head against the pillow. "Is that the way it's going to be? Food coming out of me in balls? And it feels funny coming out."

Susie drew the sheet over my gown. She pulled up a chair very close to the bed. She sat and took my hand. "Look, here's the scoop. As you well know, our system assimilates the foods we eat. It takes the nutrients from the food and eliminates the rest. What drops into your bag is your elimination. It will appear in different forms. More fibrous foods, like asparagus, mangoes, celery, onions, pea pods, these are bulky, and they tend to ball up. That's why you need to go light on them and see how your system handles them. Other foods mash up, like oatmeal and rice and pasta. Foods like bananas get pureed. Corn and peanuts, they have chaff, berries have seeds, these are not assimilated at all. They just come out in the wash, so to speak. But all foods contain liquid, and since you have no colon to handle the extraction, you'll see lots of liquid in your bag. Your body has always been a food processor, now it'll be one in a more visible way."

I don't own a food processor, but I do have a fruit juicer. I pictured it doing *its* thing. You prod the fruit into the spout, the machine whirrs, out comes the juice, pulp extracted into the little side tray. All those strings and mash in there.

"It works better for me if I think of a fruit juicer."

"There you go! And you know how the juice comes out tinted, depending on what fruit or vegetables you use? Well, the same thing happens in your body. The most alarming thing is when you have beets. We're talking red then."

"You mean if I eat beets it'll look red in the bag?"

"You bet. Watermelon too. And red Jell-O. That can be pretty scary. You've just learned that asparagus comes out green. Blueberries will be blue. Still, the body loves the color brown. As always, most foods turn to brown. Anyway, you get the picture."

I sure did. Now there was that puckery feeling again. I told Susie about it.

"That's because of the asparagus fiber. Most foods you won't even feel. Because fibrous foods are bulky, your stoma will expand to allow them to pass. Don't forget that your stoma is the end of your small intestine. And intestines expand and contract as food passes through. So what you're feeling is the movement of the intestine. You'll get used to all of that. There'll come a time when you don't feel anything at all."

"Well, right now it feels scratchy, too. Like something's pulling."

"That's probably a stitch or two around the base of your stoma. Those are dissolving stitches and they should be gone in a few weeks."

"Can things ball up so much that I get, like, stopped up?"

"Yes, so the best thing is to try foods out slowly. Chew them up well and see how they do. Drink lots of water. And listen, the most important thing is to be patient. If you have patience and are positive, you'll find that there are very few things you won't be able to eat. And just so you know, a very good remedy against getting stopped up is grape juice. Drinking grape juice keeps things moving along." Susie got up from the chair. "So, that's my lecture for now. I'll come back before dinner and show you how to empty your bag. You might need to by then."

"Hey, take your time," I said. "Take plenty of time."

True to her word, Susie came back in just when I needed her. I'd been sitting up in bed, talking on the phone, as cards and flowers arrived. Receiving them was glorious. The room was fragrant with the moist scent of blossoms. Under my gown, no more puckering, now the odd sensation of something flowing. Periodically, I laid a soft hand on the bag. I did it now. It felt warm and no longer lay flat against my belly. "I think the bag is filling," I said to Susie. "I haven't looked, but it feels like it. Also, the bag is warm."

Susie closed the door and walked up to the bed. "That's because the bag's contents are at your body temperature. That will always be the way."

"Wow. My own attached rubber bottle." I thought back to the farm, and of the rubber bottles grandma prepared for me to take to bed. Now I had one forever.

Susie set a few items on the bedside table. "Okay, time to empty that bag of yours. But first, I'll show you how it's done using a model." She produced a fresh bag—that keyhole shape, the long tail, the clip keeping it closed—and held it up for me. "What'll happen is that you'll be sitting on the toilet. The tail of the bag will be pointing down between your legs."

I pictured myself on the pot. Saw the bag hanging down, the clip at its end.

"What you'll do is lift the tail of the bag up toward you. You'll click open the clip, keeping the tail lifted and holding on to it firmly. It can be slippery, so you have to be firm." I watched her doing this. "Set the clip aside. Then turn the end of the tail over, as if you're cuffing a sock." She did this too. "Keep the end sealed by pressing with your fingers on both sides of the plastic. Remember, the bag's not empty and you don't want its contents all over the floor. So press the bag closed, then point it down and empty it into the toilet."

"Okay." I went through the steps in my mind. Lift up, unclip, cuff, keep a tight grip, empty.

"Then what you do is use toilet tissue to wipe the cuff of the tail clean." Susie was prepared. She even had a few squares of toilet paper. She dabbed them along the cuff, saying, "Wipe, wipe, wipe. Then all you do, is turn the cuff back over and re-clip. Easy as pie."

"Sure," I told her. "Easy for you to say."

"Okay, now it's your turn."

"Don't I need a pair of those gloves? You know those thin disposable ones?" My bag was half-filled with something dark green that reminded me of crank case oil.

Susie rolled her eyes. "Heavens no. You don't ever want to get persnickety with the bag and what's in it.

That would not be a good thing. You have children, right?"

I nodded.

"Think of when you changed their diapers. You didn't need gloves to do that."

"Okay. I get it."

"Good. Then let's do it."

And I did it. Not on the toilet, but in bed, because Susie thought to use that turquoise, kidney-shaped pan that's available in all hospitals. She set the pan on my lap. And, following her instructions, I emptied my first bag.

I left the hospital five days later. When I got home, a strange thing happened.

I started to cry. Jim was at sea as to how to make me stop.

• • •

A day later, my sister Anita arrived from Miami like a gale-force wind from the Atlantic. Jim went to fetch her at the airport, and when I heard the key turning in the lock, I let out a cry of joy and relief. I was lying in bed in my white, puffy robe, propped up against the pillows like a sack of old potatoes. Though it was before noon, the room was gloomy because the drapes were drawn. My eyes were red slits from all the weeping. "¡Anitía!" I cried out. My little Ani.

"¡Sandilla!" she answered, and came flying down the hall. I could feel her coming, the very air churning with her presence. I held my arms up to her and she bent down, holding me close. She smelled as she always smelled, bright floral notes touched with the scent of cedar. "Let me see you," I said, for it had been almost two years since we'd been together. Her blonde hair was held back from her forehead by a woven headband. Her dusty-blue eyes were made bluer by the navy designer suit she wore, a suit with red piping at the lapels and wrists. There were fat pearls at her neck and earlobes. "Look at you!" I said, for I had always loved the simple formality of the way she presented herself. Casual dress was not in her repertoire. I peered over the side of the bed. Sure enough. She was wearing high heels. These, red heels with pizza-slice toes. Seeing those shoes, the total reassurance they represented, set me to crying again.

"¿Qué le pasa?" Ani asked. What's the matter.

"Estoy triste." I'm sad. My incision hurt. My stitches pulled. My butt ached. I dug a tissue out of the pocket of my robe and dabbed my eyes.

Ani studied me for a moment. "Ya vamos a ver," she said at length. We'll see about that.

That old red rocking chair I'd nursed my babies in was in the room, and Ani helped me out of bed and had me sit in it, on a lambskin pad I'd been carrying around for the soft landing it provided. Me in place, she set about making things right. With a flourish, she pulled open the drapes, cracked the window for the crisp November air. She assailed the bed, pulling the sheets taut, and smoothed and smoothed, going on to vigorously fluff the pillows, her gold wrist bangles jangling merrily at every movement. Pancho Villa, my cat, had long since low-tailed it under the bed.

In preparation for her arrival, a container of baby powder sat on the dresser, for in our family it was a custom that when a person was ailing and needed to take to bed, it was sheets freshened with talcum powder that they would slip between. As if it were fairy dust, she sprinkled the bed. Generously down at the end, then less so at the top. She drew back the sheet, pulled up the fleece coverlet, and folded both back into a perfect triangle. She gave it a pat of satisfaction. "Vaya. Su cama." There. Your bed.

Just seeing it in such good order, just seeing her standing beside it all bright and good-smelling, all no-nonsense efficiency, and I started up again. "I'm sorry, I'm sorry," I blubbered. I blew my nose loudly.

Jim was in the doorway. "Since she left the hospital, she's been like that."

I nodded wetly from the rocking chair. There was plastic lying on my belly. There would forever be plastic lying on my belly. My God in heaven. What had I agreed to? Had I been out of my mind?

Ani turned to Jim. "I'm going to make soup. Do you have chicken? Onions, tomatoes, green peppers? Cilantro? Do you have that?"

We *did* have chicken, tomatoes, onions and green peppers. We also had cilantro and saffron threads and plenty of other goodies. Despite my weepy state, I'd managed to ask Jim to stock up on these, for in my family, healing could commence only after bracing bowls of homemade soup. And Ani's chicken soup could, using one of Daddy's fond expressions, cause a dead man to rise and walk another mile.

I needed Ani's soup; I needed to rise and shine.

In a little over an hour, we had *caldo de pollo con verduras* for lunch. Chicken soup with vegetables, made the Latino way. We sat at the dining room table, my lambskin pad under me. On the table lay the good placemats, the linen napkins, the silverware and china, all Ani's doing. She was still in her heels and jewelry, though she had changed into a silk blouse and jeans, jeans with a sharp crease down each leg. "Ay, Anitia, gracias," I murmured, the broth fragrant and golden in my bowl. In the broth swam rice and big chunks of chicken breast, carrot coins, and diced potatoes.

"For tonight, I'll make *tortitas,*" she announced. She ran a hand through her hair, flipping back the ends. *Tortitas* were ground chuck patties mixed with minced garlic and cilantro, with diced onions and tomatoes, the patties sautéed in butter until they made a rich brown sauce.

"*¿Tortitas con pureè de papas y petit pois?*" I asked. Tortitas with mashed potatoes and peas? My damp spirits were brightening. With my sister at my side, even for this short visit, I might start to get my gumption back. And I needed it, for soon, maybe even before bedtime, I would have to change my bag. As in peel this one off and apply a new one. In the hospital, I had watched Susie do it for me. Watched her do it twice.

Now, at home, I was on my own.

• • •

When you're an ileostomate, a bag lady or a bag man, the most important thing to learn is healthy skin maintenance. That area lying beneath the gummy round wafer that adheres the bag to the belly, that area must be protected and cared for as carefully as a baby's bottom is protected against diaper rash. In both instances, the same principle applies. Diaper rash is caused by urine sitting on the skin. Scalding, it's sometimes called. Ouch! For us ileostomates, the same irritation comes from the powerful digestive juices that are emptied into the bag and that may leak under the wafer and quickly erode the soft, tender skin of our bellies. Unlike diaper rash, which can be soothed with lotions and salves and powders, and which can be alleviated by exposure to the air, skin breakdown for bag people is tricky to treat. Lotions and powders cannot be applied and left on the skin because that would not allow for the proper adhesion needed for bag application. And no air drying is possible for us, for we have only a short window of opportunity between one bag off and the next coming on. In other words, our stomas are doing their thing, that is, dropping some form of elimination into the bag, pretty much 24/7. Without the bag in place, well . . . I'm sure you get the picture.

(For colostomates, whose stomas are on their right side and who still have their colons, skin care and elimination itself is quite different.)

Of course, I didn't know these things that first time I changed my bag myself. It was Jim who bolstered me while I did it, my sister having retired to sleep on the sofa in the den after a day of traveling, cooking and keeping my spirits buoyant.

It was after the ten o'clock news, and we were propped up in bed, Jim watching Ted Koppel on "Nightline," me studying the supplies I'd gathered around me. I had a fresh bag; to be specific, a ConvaTec ActiveLife, a one-piece drainable pouch with the Stomahesive Skin Barrier. I had a box of them, and it said so on the cover.

There are a number of different bags available. Mine was the drainable kind, that is, the one with the tail and the clip. But there are also close-ended pouches that can be detached from a faceplate that is adhered to the skin, and that need to be flushed out before they can be used again.

Unlike the bags in the hospital, the ones I had now were made of opaque plastic and not transparent, which was a good thing. Since surgery a week earlier, each time I had emptied my bag (four or five times during the day, once during the night), I had thought, There's too much visual information here. In addition to the pouch, I had a tube of Stomahesive paste, and a stack of gauze squares I would use to clean my skin and wipe it dry. To get ready, I'd moistened a few of the squares. I'd brought the kidney-shaped pan from the hospital, and I'd be using it during this first-time operation. And it was the right time to do it: my stoma had settled down for a bit. No puckery feeling, no sensation as of something flowing.

I went through the drill in my head, taking deep breaths as though I was preparing to leap off a high dive: Gently peel off the one bag, trash it, bless and thank my little stoma, clean the skin around it, pat it dry, squeeze a bead of paste around the new bag's opening, position it over the stoma, press the bag down upon the skin. To finish the process, use the little plastic clip to seal the end of the bag.

"You'll be okay," Jim said, obviously catching wind of my apprehension. "What's the worst that can happen?"

Well, the worst would be . . . what? Jim was right, this wasn't brain surgery I'd be performing. No one could die. No one ran the risk of being impaired.

I'll spare you the actual details, but suffice it to say, that give or take a few missteps, and a few anxious moments, I did the job. And Jim was by my side as I did it. He did not, I'm pleased to say, freak out when he saw my little red stoma, sitting up there so perky and businesslike on my tummy. A glorious sight, really, this thing Rob Madoff had constructed.

The support Jim gave me that night is something important. It makes such a difference to us bag wearers as we try to adjust to wearing an appliance. Jim had no problem with helping me change the bag when I thought I needed another hand. He had no problem with the contents of the bag, with the odor of these contents. It's no big deal, was his belief.

I think of the caregivers of this world, those compassionate people who tend to the ailing, the recovering, the invalid. Daily, caregivers are called to service in cleaning up all manner of bodily emissions. And though it might take a bit of getting used to, before long urine, feces, vomitus become as non-freaky to clean up as wiping a baby's face after mealtime in the highchair.

For ostomates, this kind of acceptance goes a very long way. Acceptance of this kind helps us accept our new condition, helps us become less embarrassed, less ashamed. Helps us come to believe: What's the big deal? It's only a different kind of poop.

That morning, after that debut bag-change, when I arose and went into the bathroom, there was Pancho Villa, sitting on the fluffy rug, awaiting our daily bonding time together.

I didn't quite know how to tell him that those days were gone.

• • •

My sister rolled up her sleeves while she was visiting and accomplished in ten days what I had wanted to do in the year I'd been so sick. She put order to the kitchen, refrigerator and cabinets. She cooked like a chef on fire, not only our daily meals, but enough to stock the freezer with meals for the weeks to come. She reorganized my bathroom, seeing as how I'd no longer be camping out in it, scrubbed the floor and shower stall until the tiles gleamed. Then she went at my closet and my dresser drawers, forcing me to make decisions as to what to keep, what to let go. I've been a hoarder all my life, and Ani stood at the foot of my bed in her pressed jeans, silk blouse and pizza-slice heels and lifted one item after another for me to appraise. Do you wear this? Do you like it? Does it fit? I'd gulp, trying hard to tell the truth, but she'd see the truth in my hesitations and the lukewarm way I argued her decisions.

"Goodwill. Trash. Trash," she said. "Keep. Goodwill. Keep. Trash. Keep." Each pronouncement was accompanied by a quick toss of an item onto the appropriate pile. When she finished, the "Goodwill" pile was by far the highest. The "trash" and "keep" pile came in tied.

Holding on and letting go. The neap and ebb tides of my life. For years and years, it had been hard for me to see the difference.

• • •

Days later, when changing my bag, I was shocked to find blood at the base of my stoma. Jim was at work, and I cried out to my sister, who was in the kitchen making *salpicón,* shredded beef with mint and onion and lemon juice. (The dish also calls for minced radishes, but because of their fibrous nature and in deference to me, she would omit them this time.)

Ani came rushing into the bedroom. "¿Qué, qué?"

She took one look and picked up the phone on my bedside table. "I'm calling Carlos Emilio." In less than three minutes, her husband was on the line. He was at the hospital, in Miami. Ani quickly explained the situation. I sat in bed, totally terrified. Something was terribly wrong. Like maybe my stoma was on its way to falling off. If this were true, I could not imagine what I'd done to injure it so badly. Maybe in the night, while I slept? Maybe I'd turned over too roughly? Thank God, whatever I had done had not caused pain.

"Aha," Ani said into the phone. "Aha, bueno. Aha." She presently hung up.

"¿Qué?" I asked.

"He was going into surgery, so he couldn't talk long. But he says don't worry. He says it's very common, the bleeding. That the stoma has very many blood vessels. That sometimes they bleed if you rub against something."

I lifted the gauze square I had pressed around my stoma. The gauze came away pink. There seemed to be no further bleeding. Carlos Emilio was right. I hadn't thought of it, but the stoma was red *because* of the many blood vessels.

"Carlos says just to pat it gently and the bleeding will stop. That's all you have to do. Pat it gently." She used bunched fingers, dabbing the air, to show me how.

"It's not doing it any more." My racing heart began to slow again.

"Vaya," Ani said. "Gracias a Dios."

"Thank the Lord," I echoed.

There was so much I had to learn.

• • •

A day before my sister was to leave, I began to have trouble breathing. I didn't notice it at first, but as the morning progressed, it was harder and harder to take in air. Ani and I were in the living room and I was walking toward the kitchen when I had to stop and hold on to the dining room table. I lowered my head and tried to inhale deeply, then quickly again. Then again. I turned to look at my sister who was sitting on the couch. Her eyes had gone wide, and so had mine. "Casi no puedo respirar," I managed to croak out. I can hardly breathe.

She jumped up and pulled a chair out from the table. Sat me down in it. I pressed a hand to my chest, against the poofy fabric of my robe.

"Tranquilísese," my sister said, patting my back.

My sister knows a great deal about breathing problems; she's an asthmatic and on a few terrifying occasions, she's been in respiratory crisis. "Okay," I said, trying to calm down as she instructed, and my breathing did get better, but there still was that panicky feeling, like maybe the room would run out of air. This had never happened to me before.

I sat there for a time. Taking little shallow breaths. Like a panting puppy.

Ani went into the kitchen and used the phone. I knew what she was doing. She was calling Carlos Emilio again. But this time, no such luck. Carlos was in surgery. "Where's your doctor's number," she asked, and I motioned to the side of the refrigerator. Soon, she was on the line to Rob Madoff's office.

"This is the wife of Doctor Carlos Emilio Alvarez," she began, the magic words, the open sesame, no matter where in the world. It is a true blessing to have a doctor in the family. To have a sister who can invoke the professional courtesy privileges her husband's position affords. There was an exchange of conversation, then

Ani hung up the phone. "The nurse says to take you to the hospital emergency. But if things get better, to bring you in to the doctor's office instead." She gave me a little hug. "Let's go. Now."

I rode in the back seat of the car, directing my sister on how to get to the hospital. I didn't want to sit in front where I'd have to lash the seat belt against my stoma. Because of the rush, I was still in my sleeping gown and poofy white robe, in my socks and slippers. We were on the road for perhaps fifteen minutes, when I began to feel better. I could take deep breaths and I could feel my lungs filling up when I did. "Creo que ya me'sta pasando," I confessed. I think I'm getting over it.

My sister looked at me through the rearview mirror. "¿Está segura?"

"I'm sure." The last thing I wanted was for my sister and me to have to sit for hours in an emergency room. With my mother being so sick, my sister had had to do this many times over the years.

"Then we'll go to the doctor's office," Ani said.

I protested, but my sister would have none of it. I had started this ball rolling and she was going to see the game through.

It's one thing to go to the hospital without a coat, in pajamas and robe, but another thing entirely when the destination is the doctor's office. And Rob Madoff's office at that. It was in downtown Minneapolis, in the Medical Arts Building. We were heading there during the noon hour, when lots and lots of people would be out in the streets, going to lunch.

I had my sister park in the Mar-Ten ramp, the closest parking site to the medical building. We had three blocks to walk. It was the second week of November. In the Twin Cities the air was bracing. I hooked my arm through my sister's, dropped my chin to my chest, not wanting to look up. I was living through one of my worst dreams: me in the street with hardly anything on. We hurried down the sidewalk, crossed two streets. I'm almost sure a few cars slowed down as they passed. I was stepping out of the revolving door at the front of the building, when a man caught sight of me and his expression had the question, "Is it still Halloween?" written all over it.

I took my sister's arm again and buried my head against her shoulder. Maybe it was still Halloween. In my robe, I looked like the Pillsbury Doughboy.

The Doughboy with moose-head slippers on his feet.

"Well, look at you," Rob Madoff said, when he stepped into the examining room.

I started to explain, but threw my hands up.

Because I was too befuddled to do it, Ani introduced herself, reminding Madoff that he and Carlos Emilio had talked after the operation. "I think Sandy had a panic attack," she went on to say.

"What are you panicky about?" Madoff asked, turning to me.

"I'm leaving tomorrow," Ani said, before I could answer.

"That might explain it. But let's have a look."

I crawled up on the examining table, chagrined. Why hadn't I thought of that? We could have used a brown paper bag. Breathe into it. Breathe out. But no, here I was, in downtown Minneapolis, looking like I'd just rolled out of bed.

Rob Madoff listened to my chest. I was breathing

normally now. He then checked my incision, pressed my tummy here and there. "Looks good."

I told him about the bleeding a few days before.

"Stomas'll do that," he said. "They have lots of blood vessels. You should be going back to see the enterostomal nurse, right? She'll tell you all you need to know."

I nodded. I had an appointment with Susie the day after next.

"Do you think she might need a little Valium?" Ani asked.

"That might not be a bad idea," Madoff said. "Let's try some for five days."

I wish there was something he could have given me to make me oblivious to the walk back to the car. But no, there we were, two sisters, the one walking smartly down the sidewalk in her designer heels, the other scuffling along in her Bullwinkles.

When we reached home, Ani called Carlos Emilio. She told him not to expect her on the flight tomorrow. She told him her sister would be needing her for a few more days.

• • •

In the months that ensued, I began to try to *tranquilizarme,* to do as Ani suggested when I was short of breath. *Tranquilizar,* as in, to become tranquil, to calm down. As in Marcus Aurelius's adage for good living: "The first rule is to keep an untroubled spirit. The second is to look things in the face and know them for what they are."

Knowing things for what they are. In my case, they

were that having surgery had changed my life because it had *given* me a life again. A new life, free of pain and anxiety and drug side-effects. A life free of constant reliance on the bathroom. After surgery, I was more cheerful; I had more energy; I was more productive.

And I began to turn to my faith. Not the Catholic part of me who had been banished from the Church because of my divorce and remarriage, nor the lost soul who had been told by a church deacon when I went to him for solace, "Why do you insist on being a part of a church that doesn't want you?"

I turned directly to God Himself, believing with all my heart that, despite the Church's denial, there was a deep connection between me and my Creator. I made up a little song, and I would sing it under my breath many times during the day: I love you God. I trust you God. I thank you God. A little tune to God because it's been said that when we sing to Him, we pray twice.

And I was learning what I needed to know in order to live and *thrive* as a bag lady. Susie, the enterostomal nurse, helped me on the visits I made to the hospital clinic. During those first months, not only was my life undergoing a transformation, but so was the size of my stoma. Susie showed me how to measure my little spout, how to adapt the bag opening to fit snugly around it. She helped me see that a stoma needed to make adjustments, too. That after a time, the stoma would settle down into its own particular size.

• • •

Another thing I learned was that after I healed, having sex was not going to be the problem I feared it might.

For the first few times, however, making love was a bit uncomfortable, given that my female parts had shifted somewhat after my rectum was removed. But soon all settled into position and the act felt normal again. It helped, of course, that Jim did not find my bag repugnant, that he did not consider my wearing a bag a turnoff. Still we made love when my gut was quiescent and after I'd emptied the bag. I took to covering it with those little soft shoe-shine mitts you get at hotels and which I began to collect. I slipped a mitt over the tail of the bag and up around the base. Then, I used a small, plastic paper clip to fasten the tail to the top edge.

That was ten years ago; now all manner of camouflage is available in catalogs and on the websites of ostomy suppliers. But back then, I ended up making my own little mitts. It was easy. I bought lengths of flannel fabric with cute designs: hearts, polka dots, even some with Mickey Mouse faces. I cut out rectangles to fit just right, sewed three sides together, and voilà! I'd have my own unique camouflage. And these colorful mitts proved useful in another way. I slip one over my bag each day before I pull up my panties. The mitts help to keep the plastic clip that seals the bag's tail from chafing or gouging the skin of my tummy. The mitts go into the wash. Then into the dryer, to be finally stacked up in my dresser drawer alongside my underwear.

Just another way, a sort of playful one, to make the best of a bag situation.

• • •

When I attended their meetings, the Minneapolis chapter of the United Ostomy Association helped with information on new technologies and new products on the market. I made a few phone friends at the meetings, and we frequently boosted each other with phone calls sharing tips and answering each other's questions.

One of our most common topics was the length of time between bag changes. When I first got home from the hospital, I found I needed a new bag every third day. But as I got more adept at fitting the bag opening snugly to my stoma (less risk of leaks, that way), I was able to increase that time. At the meetings, we heard talks by bag veterans, some of whom could stretch bag use to ten days and upward. Presently, almost eleven years after surgery, and being somewhat of a bag-veteran myself, I change my bag every seven, give or take a day. I can go longer, but I find that waiting longer puts my healthy skin at risk. And I keep track by writing the day of the week I made the change on the covering that backs the round wafer that's adhered to the tummy. I use a permanent marker that won't come off when it gets wet, usually a Sharpie with an ultra-fine point. Why is it necessary to do this? Because once I adjusted to having the bag, having a bag is something I rarely think about. It's like urination. I only think about it when I'm peeing, or when I need to go. So, for me, it's easy to lose track of the day I changed. Without a date to remind me, it's easy to keep the bag on much longer than I should.

Back then, the confidences we ostomates shared over the phone allowed me to see that each bag person has a unique story.

One friend, for whatever reason, had a very short stoma. She described it as almost flush to the skin. This little spout was hardly a spout. She was plagued with leakages and horrific skin irritations because of it. Another, had a problem with gas. Because, yes, while it's true that we stomates are incapable of farting, we, like everyone, have gas in our intestine and our bags inflate because of it, sometimes alarmingly. This friend found a system whereby she used a needle to prick a tiny hole at the top of her bag. She then covered it with tape. When she needed, she pulled the tape back to allow for ventilation. To that, I say, hey, whatever works for you. In my case, to expel gas trapped in the bag, I simply lift the tail upright, unseat the clip, thus allowing an opening from which the gas can escape. And I do this carefully, carefully, remembering that there's more than gas in the bag.

Diet was a never-ending topic of conversation at these meetings. What to eat? What not to eat? The causes of diarrhea, because, again, we stomates too can have this pesky malady. It manifests itself by watery elimination into the bag. And it's brought on by the same things that produce it in non-ostomates: certain drugs, food gone bad, sometimes anxiety or stress, an illness, like the flu. But it was the opposite problem that generated the most discussion. Constipation, or the bulking up of digested food that would then be difficult, or impossible, to empty. The dreaded blockage. Some people would not eat salads for fear of it. Or corn or blackberries or cabbage or Brussels sprouts. For some, popcorn was a no-no, or nuts or bananas or watermelon. I could go on and on. There was a person at one of the meetings who announced that she had the solution to never having a blockage. She only ate, she said, things that she could sip through a straw. As Dr. Phil on TV says, I'd seen more meat on antlers than what I saw on her. But she was triumphant in her announcement and—tell her what we might, that foods could be experimented with, that they could be added and subtracted as you learned their effect—there was no one in the meeting who could make her see things in a different light.

Of course, stoma blockage was everyone's fear. One phone friend had a blockage so severe that it caused her stoma to retract and she had to go back into surgery to have the problem corrected. Another person told of developing a parastomal hernia, which caused her intestine to protrude through the abdominal wall around her stoma. That, too, needed surgical intervention.

I tried to not let these stories frighten me. Instead, I saw them as cautionary tales. Hearing them, I often asked myself, what can I do to prevent that from happening to me?

And while I'm thankful to say that these major problems have never befallen me, some icky, embarrassing and frightening things have occurred, for as the crude saying goes, Shit happens.

One such time, Jim and I were in a bookstore. Luckily, it was a late Sunday afternoon and there were few patrons because the hockey playoffs were on TV. At the bookstore, I was at the "B" section, visiting the shelf on which my novel sat, right up there with novels by Elizabeth Berg. I love being in this section, because Elizabeth Berg novels are bestselling novels and readers who look for her books usually can bump into mine. So, there I was, admiring my shelf placement when I felt something wet and hot making its way south, down my leg. I called out to Jim, who was perusing the magazines, and he recognized that little high-pitched quaver in my voice that spelled BA, BA! Bag alert, bag alert!

Jim helped me duck-walk into the bathroom, which

thankfully was empty. Still, he guarded the door while I pulled my dress up and took a look. The fabulous clip was open, allowing for bag content to spill. I clicked the clip shut again, hearing that satisfying sharp sound that told me the bag's tail was sealed and went on to use half the roll of paper to clean myself up.

I learned two big lessons that day. One: Pay attention when you're closing your clip. Wait to hear that *click* that tells you it's closed. Give it a little tug to make sure that it is. ConvaTec clips are right as rain. In the years I've used them, they have never, as in NEVER, opened up on me once I've clicked one firmly into place.

Two: Fix an emergency kit for yourself and stash it in the car. Accidents can happen, not just when you're still on a learning curve, but later, too, when you're a bag-veteran. When they do, ask yourself, is this the end of the world? Am I going to die because of this? Will others die?

I don't think so.

• • •

Believe it or not, life existed beyond the bag. I was busy writing my second novel, *Bitter Grounds.* And I was a lucky girl, because Hyperion, a New York publishing house, bought the book. Even before it was finished! Another New York giant, Scribner, was publishing the paperback edition of *A Place Where the Sea Remembers* and they were sending me on a book tour.

Fifteen cities. I'd be gone for five weeks.

Can a bag lady go on such a trip, you might ask? The answer is, well, this one can. Hadn't I gone traveling in a full-body cast?

To go on a tour, all I had to do was make like a scout and be prepared.

First and foremost, The Kit. A kit to carry in my purse in case of slow leaks, or a sudden clip failure, or horror of horrors! the bag-adhesive giving way. I'd found a small makeup clutch at the mall and loaded it with the necessary items: extra bags, paste, clips, etc. In fact, when not traveling, this kit should be readily available for use when your bag needs changing. I keep mine, all stocked up, ready to use, in the bathroom closet. When bag-changing day rolls around, all I need to do is pull the kit off the shelf. No need to go pawing through boxes of supplies.

Because of the tour itinerary, I'd be spending almost as much time on a plane as I would on the ground, so packing just one small carry-on was a must. In addition, I chose a rather large purse with lots of pockets for stashing books, a notebook, makeup and bag kits, in addition to the usual.

Comfortable clothing was the only way to go. I found that jumpers were becoming my favorites. They have high waists, which provide a little fullness over the tummy and therefore make room for a filling bag. Layered with leggings and a long-sleeved T, worn with a blazer, jumpers make for smart dressing. Smart for bathroom visits, too. Especially in cramped airline bathrooms, which frequently have wet (arrrghhh!) floors. When faced with this situation, I find that it's better to lift a skirt, than to lower trousers.

Speaking of bathrooms. Here are two tips you might consider, these learned the hard way. I think I was in Seattle. I had done a reading at a bookstore and a number of us had gone to a restaurant for a late meal.

I was using the bathroom, my jumper's skirt folded nicely across my lap. I felt pretty smug that the bag-emptying was becoming old hat; I could almost do it on auto-pilot. I unclipped the bag, turned it down between my legs, then emptied half the bag's contents into . . . my panties!

And so this is my first tip: When lowering your panties, or shorts if you're a guy, make sure that you lower them sufficiently so that the back of them has not slipped between the toilet seat and the toilet cover. When this happens, they stretch out under you like a sling. Second tip, and probably the most important, when emptying your bag, even if you're at home, always, always pay attention. Leave auto-piloting to the people flying planes.

So given this little contretemps, you might want to know: How did I resolve the mess I'd gotten myself into? Well, I very carefully mopped up what I could with plenty of toilet paper. (And I do mean carefully here, because you don't want to compound the problem.) So I mopped up, blotting and blotting. Then I slipped off my pantyhose, then my soiled panties. Because I was prepared, I used the wet wipes I carried in my purse for the final tidying up. I also toted a few zippered Glad bags and I stashed my panties in one of those. Cleanup accomplished, I slipped on my panty hose. Lowered my skirt. Took three huge breaths to compose myself and, after washing my hands vigorously, went back to the table as if nothing untoward had happened.

It's what you try to do when you're a bag person: Act normal, because you are.

• • •

"Acting normally" comes with time. There's no question that, for a few months after surgery, I was superfocused on the reality that I was a BAG LADY, all caps on that descriptor. Only in the background did I think of the other things that make me what I am: daughter, sister, wife, mother, grandmother, friend, writer. Morning, noon and night it was the bag, what was in the bag, the skin under the bag, et cetera, et cetera and so forth, as the King of Siam put it in a song. I think maybe that's all I talked about, though my friends and family were too loving, too understanding to make me aware of it or worse, to chide me for it. They allowed me time and space to get reacquainted with all the things I'd always been, to make friends with the bag lady I had become.

bag lady. Term in lower case, and placed at the end of the list of who I am.

It's an important distinction, this putting our bagness at the bottom of the line. I think that women who've had mastectomies find themselves in the same position. They, as we, have lost parts of themselves. Amputation it is called. Some of them, as some of us, have had those parts replaced. They with prostheses, we with stomas and bags. But it does not serve either of us well to turn our lives into martyrdoms because of it.

We are not victims. We should not act like victims.

Bag-wearing is not our identity.

In other words, we are not our bags.

• • •

And, let's not forget a sense of humor, which, when you give it some thought, is really all about attitude, about what you choose to believe about a situation. Injecting a little levity into bad situations will certainly go a long way toward taking the sting out of them.

A sense of humor got me through another bag adventure. It happened during another book tour, this one planned by Hyperion, the publisher of my third novel, *The Weight of All Things.* I was scheduled for a reading at noon at a bookstore in San Francisco. The booksellers had prepared an excellent venue for me: chairs set up at the back of the store, a table at the front with a display of my books—all three of them, a wildflower bouquet in a vase, a little podium for me to use. A lot of people filled the seats, always a wonderful thing to see. Most had taken their lunch hour to attend, so sticking to the schedule was important.

About ten minutes to noon, I felt the unmistakable sensation that told me I was heading into trouble: the bag's adhesive was giving way. Of the three bag-emergencies (the first being the clip becoming unseated and the second, a slow leak), the adhesive pulling loose is by far the most unsettling. Unsettling, too, that I had committed the ultimate no-no: I'd left my kit in my suitcase. And my suitcase was in my escort's car. (When on tour, authors are driven from place to place by literary escorts.) Worse, he had dropped me off and then parked the car a good hike away. It was noon, after all, in San Francisco. Most choice parking spots had been taken. Nevertheless, when I confessed my dire predicament, my angel escort dashed off to retrieve the suitcase. Still, all serious repairs would have to be made after the reading, not before. All I could hope to accomplish in the ten minutes before the reading would be some kind of Band-Aid repair.

Which gave me an idea. I dashed up to the information desk. "I'm the author doing the reading," I said, "but a bit of an emergency's come up. A sort of medical emergency."

The bookseller's eyes widened. "Are you okay?"

"Do you have any duct tape?" I asked. "I can fix it with duct tape."

"Duct tape?" Her eyes went even wider, as if her mind were whirling around trying to land on a medical condition that duct tape might fix.

"Yeah, you know 'duck tape'? That silvery tape that everyone pokes fun at?" I had remembered that at one of the meetings I'd attended, someone had told a story about fixing a bag with this kind of tape. "That stuff will stick to anything," that person had said.

The bookseller rummaged under the counter; she opened a few drawers, pawed through them, but came up empty.

Under the layers of jumper, shirt, slip and panties, I could feel the added tug of more adhesive pulling away. "I really need some tape," I said.

"Hold on." She turned and disappeared into a back room. Time was ticking away. There were people in chairs, waiting for an author to read to them.

"Look!" the bookseller said, coming triumphantly through the door again. "But there's not much left on the roll."

"You're an angel," I said, rushing toward the bathroom with my prize.

In the stall, I peeled away the layers to assess the damage. It was not good. I cleaned up what was needed, then I used the tape (it indeed sticks to anything) to secure the bag against my tummy. I used—a mile?—of toilet paper to lay over the bag for possible soaking-up purposes. I tell you, that extra room provided by my high-waisted jumper came in very handy. (Please note that I don't recommend this method of repair. Using Duct Tape can seriously damage the skin.)

Thus, temporarily repaired, I strolled into the reading area right on time.

After the reading, after the Q&A, after chatting with a few lingerers, I dug into my suitcase, which my escort had kindly and hastily fetched, and used the staff's private bathroom to make the best of a really, really bad bag situation.

Of course, I let the booksellers and my escort in on what was happening to me, for they were very curious as to the cause of the emergency. It is not a problem for me to speak about these things. I don't believe we bag people should be secretive about our situation. Our situation is not something to hide. On the other hand, it's not information we're obliged to volunteer. I'm reminded of Lyndon Johnson, who used to pull down the top of his trousers to show the incision from his hernia operation. Hello! Give us all a break.

The bottom line is this: when the occasion merits it, speak up. If not, keep mum. When people ask "How are you?" you don't have to pull up your shirt, peer down at your bag, and say, "Let me check." In other words, the question should not be taken literally and then answered as such. The majority of people don't really wish to learn what ails you.

• • •

Going on tour provided me with an unexpected benefit. Traveling around the country took me, on a number of occasions, to Miami to visit my parents, my sister and her family, as well as to Los Angeles and Tucson, where Jon and Chris lived. At these times, I forwent the escort and hotel accommodations, preferring instead to stay with my family. Sitting with them in living rooms and at tables over dinner, I slowly opened up and spilled out the past, talking about subjects that mattered to me. It was a revelation to find that when I spoke the truth, when I finally divulged the why of things, the world did not come tumbling down. When I was honest, my family did not turn away from me as I had feared they might.

In my fourth novel, *Night of the Radishes,* a minor character makes a major pronouncement about these common silences affecting so many families. Her name is doña Clarita and she's a Mexican healer, much like nana, in El Salvador, had been. She says to Annie Rush, my main character, a Minnesotan: "A true story is a story, no matter what language is used to convey it. And it's not so much the story's content that's important. What's important is that it be told. That it be brought up from the heart, pushed out by the breath, released into the air. Freed. Freed to mingle and collide with all the other freed stories permeating the air around us. It's where stories belong, outside us, not trapped and calcified within, weighing us down like sea anchors."

In my life, there had been so much weighing down by stories left untold. All of them hardening into stone inside my gut.

• • •

I began honoring my own sacred stories by creating a personal altar in my studio, a place I'd acquired using money I'd made from writing those other stories that had collected in "the soft-waxed area inside (me) where all that had touched down had left a soft impression." I'd found this wondrous sentence in a slender, perhaps now out-of-print, book titled *Side Glances: Notes on the Writer's Craft,* by John V. Hicks. This concept moved me so deeply when I first read it, and my continued musings about it helped me to see that such a place had indeed, and throughout my life, existed around my heart. Over time, extraordinary and seemingly ordinary experiences had collected, layer upon layer, into this pool of cooling wax. It is here I dip my pen when starting to write or tell a story.

This studio of mine had been in fact my neighbor's apartment. Jim and I live in a condo, and when the opportunity arose, we bought the small one-bedroom next to ours, knocked an opening in the wall, put in a door and, praise the heavens above, my own sacred space was created. It's a wonderful thing to be so close to home that I can leave one place in my pajamas and never have to climb into a car to start writing. The studio has a living room with fireplace, a summer screened-in porch off that, a dining room, a bedroom, one bathroom, plus full kitchen and laundry facilities. In all, nine hundred or so square feet with a delightful view of a back yard filled with big high trees and a little pond with a waterfall tucked in a corner. All in all, it is a miracle.

Before I moved all my writing stuff over, I took my time in making the place entirely my own. Virginia Wolf would be pleased, I'm sure of it.

To start things off, I painted the walls using a faux finish, an ochre colorwash in the living and dining rooms, brick red in the kitchen, burnt orange in the bathroom, mossy green in the bedroom. I had new carpet laid, white Berber, which offsets the walls nicely.

In the living room I set up my computer on an L-shaped desk spacious enough to hold the printer and all my papers and piles of books. There's an old comfy sofa against the wall, a number of bookcases so crowded with books that all the shelves are bowing. The walls are covered with photos and art. The tops of the bookshelves hold all manner of things: sculptures, statues, lamps. The place is so loaded with what I call art, that if something new catches my eye, I have to give plenty of thought to what would have to come down for it to go up.

I've converted the dining room into an altar room. In so doing, I've adopted a Latino tradition in which a place is set aside in a home to honor God and the ancestors. Because my loved ones are buried in various far-off locations, I use the altar as my own family graveyard.

My altar is made from an old Hoosier cabinet, the kind that long ago graced farmhouse kitchens. I bought mine twenty-five years ago. It is a tall, wide piece of furniture comprising a three-door cupboard set upon a base. The base has a set of side drawers (one served as a flour bin with a sliding cover) and a two-door cabinet with wire shelves, this topped with a sheet of white galvanized tin. Many a farm wife kneaded dough upon a surface such as this, and I sometimes think of the woman who must have stood at mine. I think of her strong hands working at what would be transformed into the family's daily bread. I think of her dreaming there, much like grandma must have done, her hands and fingers, her body, surrendering to the rhythmic rolling out and folding in. I can hear the dull sound her fist makes as periodically she punches the dough into compliance. Was she a happy woman standing there?

Was the life she was living the whole of her heart's desire?

Being a dreamer, too, as I go about my day, I often ask myself, Who once stood upon this spot? Who sat on this church pew, this station bench? Who lived in this house? Slept in this room? Who ambled along this sidewalk? Crossed this street? These transitory thoughts some might find odd, but in my case, I draw comfort from the thought of how we are connected to so many people, invisible though they may be. If we could but see these entities beyond our sight, we would know with certainty that we are not alone. In any case, I bought a Hoosier cabinet and thereby purchased with it stories I imagine and invent.

Which brings to mind the memory of an old trunk I purchased in Saint Louis when the kids were small. It was a flat-topped trunk, just the kind to convert into a coffee-table. I found it in an antique store and the owner gave me a good price because it was locked shut and the key had long been lost. As I pushed and pulled the trunk out to the car, its hefty weight had me dreaming of precious loot trapped inside. Gold coins? Jewelry? Fine art?

Because I didn't want to destroy the ornate brass key plate, it took me a week to pick the lock. It was a metal nail file that finally did the trick.

When I lifted the lid, I discovered this: burnt-wood boxes for scarves and gloves; hand-embroidered handkerchiefs, lacy blouses, a silky slip; a small leather purse; a beaded bag. There were letters with two-cent stamps and postcards with one-centers, all postmarked in the 1920s. There were dozens of valentines, some from Ina and Imogene, some from Wilson and Carl, all addressed to Helen Miller. One card had scalloped edges and featured an accordion-folded heart that popped out when opened and was, most sincerely, from Tashido Sonada. In addition, there were granny glasses and a lorgnette. A collection of thimbles. Wrapped inside yellowed tissue paper laid a square of silk, an inky background sprinkled with red and blue flowers.

After almost forty years, I've kept Helen Miller's treasures because fragments of her stories are contained in them, and I have honored that.

I think of my family. Objects passed from hand to hand. Stories told, others not talked about. Dear friends and acquaintances recount stories of their own. In public places, behind walls and doors, voices rise. Stories float up and are deposited into the trunk of our collective unconscious. We have only to coax a lock to set the stories free.

• • •

Down in Miami, another story was unfolding. My mother was ailing, big-time, and my father, Ani and I were very much on top of things. The list of Mami's complaints, her medications, her "procedures," was so long that Daddy had written and printed out a report that he'd hand out to healthcare providers when they began to ask their questions. "If your mother were a soldier," he often told us, "she'd have a chest-full of medals and ribbons for all she's been through." You could say that again. She suffered from rheumatoid arthritis, diabetes, osteoporosis and heart disease (she'd had a double-bypass). She'd had breast cancer and had endured a double mastectomy. She was anorexic (at one time her weight fell to 69 pounds) and had developed such severe food phobias that she'd only open her mouth to an ounce or so of white chicken meat, a tablespoon or two of boiled rice and half of a banana. Before she'd have the banana, however, she insisted that it be de-seeded. A banana de-seeded? Yes. All those little dark spots in them had to go. In 1998, you could add paranoia to the list. There was a battalion of ants in the living room, largartijas, lizards, as well. When she went into the bathroom, she donned a set of those throwaway rubber gloves. Afterward, at the sink, she'd scrub her naked hands with a soft brush. Over and over, the scrubbing. Needless to say, the lack of proper nutrients was now affecting her brain function. On then to specialists who prescribed anti-depressants and anxiety medications. For a period of months, and after she returned home from yet another hospital stay, she was placed on tube-feeding, and Daddy became an expert at hooking her up to the line and keeping track of the monitor readouts. He was also now an expert at keeping her blood sugar in check: pricking her, adjusting the insulin doses and injecting her.

That my sister and her husband lived nearby meant everything. Ani was at my parents' beck and call; she fixed nourishing meals for them, found caregivers when they were needed, went shopping when lists were provided. Because Carlos Emilio was a physician, test results were always only hours away, private hospital rooms became speedily available, doctor friends of his came out to my parents' house when a crisis arose and a quick response was needed.

In the fall of '98, such a crisis occurred. Mami tried getting out of bed alone and slipped down the side of the bed to the floor. It happened in a flash, before Daddy could reach her, and the movement, slow and gentle as it was, broke her back so riddled with osteoporosis.

At the news, I flew down immediately. I stayed for almost a month. In that time she had a two-step spinal surgery: She was opened from the back, where a titanium cage was implanted around the broken sections of her spine. A week later, she was opened from the front and this cage was reinforced with pieces carved from one of her ribs.

Before she was wheeled into the first procedure, and because her chances to survive were slim (she weighed 72 pounds), she made us promise that if she didn't make it, we would bury her next to Susanita. Though it meant flying her body to Washington, D.C., we promised her we would. "Of course, Mami. Of course," we each said to her.

But a miracle occurred. Mami survived the carnage of her surgery and went on to live almost another year. When she did die, in October 1999, her death was so sudden (a drastic imbalance of electrolytes) that arrangements could not be made in time for her body to be transferred to Washington.

Daddy was bereft. He'd lost the love of his life, though he'd struggled so hard to keep her alive. He'd prayed ceaselessly, his silent clamorous requests sent up to God in spirals of incense he burned on his window ledge. The fact that we'd had to bury Mami in Miami and not next to Susanita, as we'd promised, added to his grief.

But I had an answer for Daddy. I promised that after the shock of Mami's death had passed, I'd make a trip to Washington and have Susana exhumed. I'd then bring her remains to Miami. "When it's your time to join Mami," I said, "I'll bury Susanita with you and then Mami and Susanita will be reunited again."

Daddy's sad eyes had lighted up at the suggestion. My aching heart had cheered a bit as well.

• • •

The loss of a mother is a partial loss of the self. It was for me. Her death cast me adrift, for she took with her her memory, both spoken and untold. She took all she might have divulged about herself, about me, for from the moment she passed, from the moment I watched her face soften and ease as she took death's hand, as she grasped her Susanita's, a myriad of questions I might have asked descended on me like a sudden sleeve of rain. With her went all that possibility.

It's often said that life is a circle, but I see it as a spiral, that ancient symbol of unity and multiplicity, of wisdom and eternity. A spiral, concentric swirls where all is a continuum. I think about how our own DNA is represented by a helix, that lovely ascending spiral. The circles upon circles of code it contains. The stored memories, the stories. Stories captured by the orbit of our eyes. Stories reverberating in the volute shell of our ears. Stories imprinted in the whorls at our fingertips. When we speak, are we not surrendering stories by the pursed circle of our lips?

When Mami died, her stories went with her, and though I'd been too self-centered to ever ask, all she knew and felt about Susana was lost to me as well.

• • •

To recover a few memories, I agreed to travel to El Salvador some months later. My brother-in-law was making a trip to do pro bono work at a hospital there, and he and my sister invited me to accompany them. One of the first things I did after I settled in was visit the house on Avenida Olimpica, the house from which, at fourteen, I was catapulted into the world.

It was a Sunday when I arrived, the day warm and breezy. As I drew near to my familiar address, I noted with dismay how the neighborhood had turned commercial. Pulling up to the curb, I noted that my house was now a computer science school: Escuela Superior de Informática. At the top of the drive, beside the door, stood a guard. He wore a gray uniform, the trouser legs tucked deep into tall boots. From his attire alone, I couldn't make out what he was: police? guardia nacional? private security? He held a rifle almost casually across his chest, and for some odd reason this cavalier stance gave me hope I might talk him into allowing me entrance. As I went toward him, I bowed my head to allow him his importance. "Buenos días, Señor Oficial," I said. To my delight, when I reached the door, it was open and swung wide. There the familiar tiles of the small foyer. Beyond that, the living room making a turn to the left.

He stared at me. He appeared to be in his forties. His narrow face looked haggard, but his dark eyes shadowed what he'd lived.

I pointed to inside. "A long time ago, this was my house, Señor."

He said nothing. As if his thoughts were printed in a cartoon-bubble above his head, I could see what he was thinking: The little gringa speaks Spanish. What does she want? Is there some gain for me in what she wants?

I continued: "I lived here when I was a girl. I've come

all the way from the United States to visit it again." My voice had a tremble in it, which I did not have to invent. Before I could be dissuaded, I poked my head inside. Beyond the doorframe and immediately on the left was the narrow hall off of which was the guest bathroom. A man came out of the bathroom. He was tugging up his pants. He gave a start when he saw me, and I pulled back, afraid I'd ruined everything. "Can I please go in?" I asked the guard behind me. The guard shook his head.

The man inside came to fill the doorway. The butt of a revolver poked out of his waistband. Not letting the sight of it discourage me, I decided to tell a story. "Señor, when I was a girl, this was my house." I didn't wait for a response, but stepped boldly through the door and around him. I pointed to a spot on the foyer floor. I went to stand upon that spot. "See this? This is the place where I received my first kiss. I was fourteen." Mi primer beso, is what I said.

The information disarmed both men.

"It's true. I was standing right here when my boyfriend kissed me."

At my confession, the bathroom-man gave a little laugh. The guard smiled.

I said, "It was the first time he kissed me, but it was also the last."

The men laughed grandly then, so I took it as a sign and strode all the way in.

• • •

It was only me and the guard and his rifle. The bathroom-man remained in the doorway. I understood this presence of security: since the war, gangs of thieves and muggers roamed El Salvador causing chaos of a different sort. In the living room, I turned a circle and took in my past. I stood on that sea of red tiles cross-hatched by white grouting. The very tiles over which I'd stepped so long ago. If I lowered an ear to them, would I catch my old comings and goings?

Though the tiles were the same, the walls and windows appeared to have shrunk over the years. The house was tiny compared to the way it had lived in my memory. The glass doors that led out to the patio were there, but the patio itself was gone. No more flagstone on which to dance passionately in stockinged feet. No little pool; no bright sun. Gone was the mauve bougainvillea spilling over the back wall. Gone the hovering, darting hummingbirds. The area had been enclosed and converted into a classroom. Rows of long tables were topped by a dozen computer monitors and screens.

The wide S-shaped staircase that led to the second floor was still as grand as I remember it. When my mother splattered brick-colored paint on white sailcloth to fashion new draperies, she'd had the staircase painted a deep rich green. The color had contrasted strikingly with the floor tiles. But that showiness was also a thing of the past. I climbed the stairs slowly, my hand slipping over the metal hand rail that I'd held as a youngster. Back then, I'd swish up the stairs, descend them in a rush, or in a slow dramatic glide, whatever best fit the occasion.

At the top of the stairs and a few steps across the landing stood my bathroom. A sign on the door read "Damas." I looked in and it was 1955 again: the same shower stall with the green speckled tile. It looked so cramped, it was a wonder I'd never felt claustrophobic when I took long soaking showers. The same mirror crowned the vanity: round-topped and etched with garlands of flowers around the edges. I looked into the glass, expecting to see a smooth young face, brown hair pulled severely into a ponytail. In the mirror, I could see the guard behind me. He stood on the landing, the strap of his rifle now hooked over his shoulder.

The door to my bedroom was a few steps from the bathroom. It was locked, but there was a window halfway down I could peer through. The walls held whiteboards; small desks took up most of the space. I erased these from my sight, picturing instead my old dresser with the bombé legs, my bookcase, my bed with its pink chenille spread. That bed had rested under a low window and late at night, I'd lie on my stomach and look out into the dark, up the street where the statue of el Salvador del Mundo seemed to float in an upsweep of illumination. I remembered lying there one night. I was almost fifteen. A friend's mother had just committed suicide. It was he who found her and cut her down from the rope. Back then, my mind swirled with that terrible event. With the added knowledge that soon I'd be leaving my world behind. Daddy had given the order: Off I'd go to grandma and grandpa's farm. Off I'd go to become Americanized.

Back then, I knew that the one event—that is, the suicide—had not caused my father to send me away, but somewhere in my mind, perhaps I had linked these two things. When in rehab at Hazelden, I came to understand things about myself I had never before acknowledged. Such as leaving home at a tender age. It was as if Daddy had slipped a loving noose around my neck. Buried deep in the tangle of my psyche was Mami. I had wanted Mami to find me. Wanted her to cut me down from that rope before I was gone.

I stepped over to my parents' bedroom. Its door was also locked, but it had a window in it as well. I knew it was there that I'd been heading all along. To that space that had once held my parents' marriage bed, my mother's dreams, my father's aspirations. There, to my left, was the closet where Mami's strongbox had resided. I pressed my head against the glass.

She was frequently ill, even back then. Some days, she'd lie in bed and languish, a compress smelling sharply of Vicks VapoRub across her forehead. A servant would bring a tray of something bland that would not upset the stomach. Daddy was away. He'd roared off in his orange Beetle to yet another job to keep the quality of our life afloat.

I felt the tears slip down my cheeks. I fished inside my purse for a tissue. The guard was beside me and his expression had softened. He reached out a hand, then immediately let it drop. I was touched by this spontaneous show of kindness, aborted as it was. I wiped my tears. "Mi mamá acaba de morir. En los Estados Unidos." I said. My mother just died in the United States. "Su muerte fué muy difícil." Her death was very hard.

• • •

Upon returning home, and in the months that followed, I made arrangements for Susana's exhumation at the Washington National Cemetery in Suitland, Maryland. The director and I set aside a day in the spring. A day when perhaps the cherry trees would be blooming.

When the time arrived, Jim and I flew to Washington

from Minnesota; my father from Miami. Anita wouldn't be joining us, for one of her daughters was scheduled to deliver a baby that week. To tell the truth, I'd prayed that Daddy would stay home as well, for I knew the trip would test the limits of his grief. Coming to Washington was to arrive at ground zero, to the place where he'd met his beloved, fallen in love and married. I voiced my concern to Daddy, but he could not stay away, he said. "It's what Martita would have wanted."

I'd booked a hotel in Foggy Bottom, a spacious suite to accommodate the three of us. Jim and I were there a few days before Daddy's arrival. Though it was early April, the weather was raw. That first night the wind picked up and the sky opened up and spit snow. I pulled a chair up to our hotel window, leaned my head against the cool pane and watched the traffic crawl along on Pennsylvania Avenue. The hotel banners whipped in the wind, their metal ends clanking against their poles. Inside my heart, the same kind of disquiet.

The next morning dawned fresh and glistening, the snow washed away by a gentle, middle-of-the-night rain. We had an appointment with the cemetery director and with the priest who'd be officiating the disinterment the next day. After breakfast, when Jim and I hailed a cab to take us there, God dropped Mr. Walter Wilson and his town car directly into our lives.

He was a black gentleman who sported a professional driver's cap and a thin dark tie. His vehicle was spotless. When I told him where we were heading, he made no comment as I thought he might; after all, how many fares ask to be transported to a cemetery? He simply delineated the route for us: we'd go up Pennsylvania to Southern Road. Cross the Anacostia River, turn left on

Suitland, drive up to the top of the hill. The drive would take about thirty minutes, he informed us. His directions were so precise I asked if he'd been there before. "I'm familiar," was his response. He agreed to wait at the cemetery and then bring us back.

We struck up a conversation as we made our way. Mr. Wilson had been in the "transportation business" for near forty-five years. He enjoyed time spent on the road, weaving his car around so much significance: the grand monuments, the magnificent edifices. He enjoyed pointing these out to his fares, he said. He enjoyed telling stories as he did.

His admission prompted one of my own. I told him what we were up to. "Tomorrow we'll be exhuming my sister's body," is how I put it. I then went on to tell him the whole story. Jim sat silently beside me, taking it in for yet another time.

"Why, I've never heard of such a thing," Mr. Wilson said, when I grew silent. It occurred to me then to ask. "Do you think you could drive us there tomorrow? Could you wait for us, and then drive us back. My father will be coming in tonight. It'll be just the three of us tomorrow."

Mr. Wilson lifted his cap and repositioned it on his head. "I could most certainly provide you with transportation," he said, catching my eye through the rearview mirror.

"Oh, I'm so glad," I said, relief washing over me, for incredulously this one detail had escaped all my planning.

Mr. Wilson looked back at me again. "Pretty powerful what you folks are doing," he said. "Pretty powerful, it surely is."

• • •

We rose early the next morning. I'd made coffee in our kitchenette and Daddy, Jim and I, cups in hand, stepped silently around each other. My father was wearing his light-blue cotton robe. He'd cinched it at the waist over his boxer shorts and T-shirt. His white stork legs poked down into corduroy slippers. Somehow, with his graying hair and that wide, open face of his, he resembled Pope John Paul. When Mami was dying, he'd kept the dawn vigils beside her, looking just like that. Mami had lain mute and still in the hospital bed we'd brought into her room in the apartment. We'd long removed her wig and what little hair she had had soaked into ringlets. This excessive and constant perspiration was a consequence of diabetes, just one of her maladies. She had weighed less than seventy pounds and so she was a tiny, broken bird, gazing up at her husband who looked like the Pope. Daddy had pinned soft eyes on her, his cheeks damp with tears, his big hand gently patting his darling's hands, gnarled by arthritis and mounded like kindling over her chest. "My little bride," he'd whisper, sighing deeply. My heart ached at the sight of him then. It ached for him in Washington, where everywhere he turned, where all his eyes rested upon, carried haunting memories.

We went down to the hotel lobby in anticipation of Mr. Wilson's arrival. Precisely on time, he pulled up in his long black car. We were a huddled trio, somberly dressed, stepping out to meet it. Mr. Wilson came around the car to help us in. I was stunned by the sight of him. He was dressed for a cemetery service in an elegant black suit, starched white shirt, polished, tasseled shoes. The sight of his compassionate respect touched me almost to tears. He greeted us, informing us that traffic was a mess because of a major demonstration against the World

Bank, but not to worry, he added. He had formulated an alternate route that would get us to the cemetery on time. I was holding Jim's hand. I told myself to relax.

The new route was providential. It took us down East Capitol Street, and when we turned onto it, Daddy exclaimed, "I used to live here!" He pointed to a section of row houses. "In that one there." Gnarly brownstones. Bumped-out bay windows. Wide steps leading to carved wooden doors.

Mr. Wilson pulled over at the curb. "There's time for a stop," he said.

Daddy took a memory trip: In 1939 he lived here with three buddies. The Capitol was only a few blocks away. He worked there as a page for Senator Clark from Idaho. Not far was the streetcar. Three times a week, he'd ride it all the way to Georgetown to see his Martita. Sitting up front, beside Mr. Wilson, Daddy shook his head. "Oh, well, that was a long time ago."

Surprisingly, we got around the downtown congestion with ease. Soon we crossed the Anacostia River and proceeded up Southern Road. Daddy craned his head right and left, taking everything in. Presently, he asked Mr. Wilson, "Have you heard of Fort Davis Street?"

"It's just up ahead. We still have time; I can turn in."

Mr. Wilson made a left when we reached it. Daddy directed him to a particular row of apartments. "This is where we lived," he said, pointing to one of them.

The place was two stories of plain red brick. It had a landing, a front entrance with a screen door, a narrow window at the left. The street was deserted. Nothing appeared to move behind window or screen. Daddy stepped out of the car and I followed, leaving the others behind. We crossed the sidewalk and stood there, looking up the front walk at the apartment.

"Did I live here, too, Daddy?"

"You and Susanita lived here inside your Mami's tummy. After you were born, and when you left the hospital, you lived here for a few months. Then we moved into our little cottage in Green Meadows."

I felt the tears brimming. This street, Susana, these trees, this walk we once called our own. That landing, that screen, that door, were ours, too. It dawned on me then, that it was here, on that landing, that a harried cemetery salesman once talked a young newly married man into making an investment he could ill afford. "This is where you bought those burial policies, isn't it, Daddy?"

He nodded, silent for a moment. "The hearse carrying your sister's body went past here. Down the street and up the hill."

Standing on that spot that still contained my family's past, grief was made new. It was May 3, 1941, again and, miles and miles away, I was one month and eight days old. I lay in a hospital incubator, feeling the loss that would forever weigh my heart, that had forever dimmed the lights of my mother's world.

I slipped an arm through Daddy's and he took my hand and softly patted it. Like he used to do with Mami's hand. "I want to tell you something, honey. Something I've never told anyone before. Something that happened the day your sister was buried. Something, that after it happened, your Mami and I never spoke about."

I steadied myself for added grief.

"That day Martita and I rode in the hearse while the others trailed behind in their own cars. The hearse had a long bench-seat and we sat on it, Susanita's casket resting between us. It was a small wooden casket, and it fit easily on the seat. It was covered in white pleated silk and edged in satin ribbon. It was a pretty thing, with etched silver handles on both ends." Daddy spoke and I listened, both of our eyes set upon the apartment and its faded brick facade, the window and doorframes in need of fresh paint.

"The casket lid was not nailed down, but secured with two wide ribbons that were set in the top and pulled down over the side and tied in bows around two shanks."

I took in a quick breath, held it against what would come next.

"We'd been traveling maybe three, four minutes, our hands resting on the casket, our fingers laced together, when your mother pulled her hand away from mine. In a moment so swift it's always seemed like a blur, she untied the ribbons and raised the casket's lid. She reached into the casket and scooped Susana up. 'I never got to hold her, Jimmy,' your mother said. 'I never once got to hold her.' Tears sliding down her face, your mother held her baby in a fierce embrace against her breast."

"Ay, Mami," I muttered, a scene from my novel *Bitter Grounds* flashing through my mind and clutching at my heart. Mercedes, one of the main characters, loses her first child a few days after his birth. She can't bear to let him go (*How can I give him up?* she asks herself.), so she sits outside her hut under the laurel tree, her tiny boy clutched against her breast until he turns to stone.

This scene I had invented not knowing what my mother had endured. It's what happens when I write if I'm very lucky. The cosmic way one story will connect with a larger one. Somewhere in my very bones, I'd known my mother's story even though she'd never spoken it. It pained me beyond measure to think of her reading my book and coming upon that passage, the old scars of grief broken open again.

Tears slipped down my face as Daddy continued. His voice was shaky. "For a time, I let her hold the baby. Then, when we got near the cemetery, I had to pry Susanita from your mother's arms. I laid the baby back into the casket and refastened the lid. All I could think to say was, 'Our baby's in heaven now, Martita. She's in heaven now.'"

I rested my head against my father's arm. I felt him shudder back his own tears. "They're both in heaven now."

It took us a moment to compose ourselves. When we did, we turned back toward Mr. Wilson's car, parked there by the curb, waiting for us.

• • •

When we arrived at the cemetery, the grave had been unsealed. The damp earth it contained was mounded beside it and covered with a tarp that looked like grass. The opening of the grave itself was overlaid in the same manner. Our little group stood around it, heads bowed, hands bunched together. The priest spoke of the grief of separation, the joy of reunion. In celebration, he provided us with Holy Communion.

I read a prayer my sister Ani had sent, a prayer about an angel transcendent, an angel that lights, that rules, that guides.

I had written a few words for my mother, and I

addressed her formally then: "Mami, what we do here today was ever your heart's desire, but you passed on before we could make it come true. Being mortals, the fact weighs down our hearts. But thankfully, Mami, we believe in the communion of saints and we find comfort in the knowledge that you are here with us today, watching over these proceedings. We believe that you've now joined Susana and all our loved ones gone before. Though you are unseen, we believe that today you are all beside us, that you all are giving thanks." Despite my words, swirling inside me like wild wind were grief and regret and not a small amount of anger at what I've lacked, what I've missed.

After a moment, the tarp was removed and the grave exposed, revealing a yawning square of reddish clay. At its bottom, clumped, damp earth rested on a length of cardboard. A groundskeeper climbed down into the grave and carefully brought up the remains and set them on the grass.

I was at Daddy's side. "Dust to dust," he said under his breath.

I knelt and laid my hand on the little mound that was cool and damp against my palm. There is nothing left of you, Susana. Wherever you have been, here in this scarred soil or away from here, locked in our mother's heart and in her sad memory, you've been always in my marrow, my blood. You have been the angel watching over me.

The funeral director carried over a boxy bronze urn lined with heavy plastic. I withdrew my hand as the groundskeeper scooped damp earth into the urn. Two pounds of bone and flesh absorbed and transformed over time. Only Susana's essence was captured there and that alone was enough. There were still, however, a few evidences of what this earth contained: two fragments of coffin wood and a pair of silver handles that were attached to it. When all was in the urn, the plastic liner was sealed and the urn's lid replaced and screwed down at each corner. The groundskeeper handed the urn to the funeral director. The funeral director handed the urn to me.

It was surprisingly heavy, but I grasped it firmly. I smiled wanly at Daddy, tears clouding my eyes, tears clouding his. "It is done, Daddy," I said.

He shook his head, as if to clear a memory. He began to recite the Hail Mary, Mami's favorite prayer. Jim and I and the priest joined him. When we finished, Daddy added the angel prayer that Mami prayed frequently each day in Spanish. The prayer ended with the words: No tengas miedo. Ni de tu sombra te espantes. Do not fear. Allow not even your shadow to frighten you.

Amen, amen, I said, as Mami always did.

We crossed the lawn toward the town car parked at the edge of the cemetery lane. Mr. Wilson stood beside the door, somberly attentive.

My arms around the urn, I pressed Susana against me. It was decided I would keep her with me until Daddy passed away. We'd have a year and a half together, but this I couldn't guess. Would never have imagined Daddy's horrifying end in September, 2001.

• • •

I carried Susana's urn back to Minnesota in my carry-on backpack. The cemetery had provided a certificate of the urn's content, so I had little trouble getting through security. To my relief, the X-ray personnel handled the urn with respect and did not insist on opening it. "I'm sorry for your loss," the inspector said, when he waved us through. And I'm happy for my gain, I thought to myself, for this was a reunion I never would have imagined. After takeoff, I placed my sister's urn on my lap, next to the window. "Susana's a traveling girl now," I said to Jim.

Back home again, I placed her at the forefront of my altar. The sight of the urn and what it represented was never lugubrious, nor even sad. It was, instead, an affirmation, a verification that indeed she had existed. Every day, laying a hand on the proof of it, I'd say a little prayer over her. As Mr. Wilson had stated, "it was a powerful thing."

That fall I received a call from Michael Collier, the Bread Loaf director, inviting me to join the 2001 faculty list. Without hesitation, I said yes. The next summer, I would return to Vermont, to the place where I'd heard the harsh words that had almost caused me to stop writing. To return as an instructor there, would be a miracle of sorts.

A second honor came on the heels of the first. That winter, much to my delight and amazement, I was awarded the Knapp Chair in Humanities from the University of San Diego, and invited to teach two courses in creative-writing. My residency would start in January 2001 and end in June. I, of course, readily accepted. Before long Jim and I were on the road, driving away from cold, cold Minnesota and meandering our way through Kansas, Nebraska, Oklahoma, Texas, New Mexico and Arizona. A week later, we pulled up to the house we'd rented in San Diego. It was January 7th.

For the duration of the trip, I'd wedged Susana's urn between a suitcase and the back window, thus providing her with a splendid view of the country we passed.

It had been less than a year since her disinterment and already she had traveled the breath of the country. She was indeed a traveling girl.

• • •

After Mami passed away, Daddy moved in with Anita and Carlos Emilio. Their place in Coral Gables is one of those grand, century-year-old houses with plenty of room and a back patio splendid with live oaks. Daddy took the east wing of the house, a suite of two rooms and private bath. It was perfect for him. He used one of the rooms for a den and an office, spending most of his day working on a memoir I'd urged him to write some years before, when his mother, my Grandma Hazel, had died and I was driving him to Missouri for the funeral.

During the trip, Daddy told me stories. They were all about separation and longtime regret. He had left the farm and his mother's side at seventeen, when he joined the Navy. Until her death, sixty plus years later, if you added the time he'd spent with her it would not have amounted to more than half a year. He'd made maybe five trips to Missouri. Stayed a week or so each time. Grandma herself had done some traveling, coming from Missouri for a few visits. Then that one time, when she and Daddy had met in Washington, D.C., and he'd had the pleasure of showing his patriotic mother all the city's museums and monuments. But for the most part, over the years, grandma had stayed put while her son went wandering.

Driving toward that final encounter, I urged my father on. Tell me about when you were in the Naval Academy, Daddy. Tell me about that time in the Chiapas jungle when you were searching for a source of penicillin. Tell me about your gladiola plantation, about building a stretch of the Pan American Highway, about when you started Sun Airlines down in the Ozarks. Tell me, Daddy. Tell me, tell me. After the funeral, and when he was back in Miami, I wrote him a long letter thanking him for that precious time we had spent corralled in my car, the road rolling steadily beneath us, his stories leaving their impression in that soft-waxed area of my heart. In the letter, I also suggested he write the stories down. I even included a list of topics he might consider.

And so he had considered my request and begun. *The Recollections of Jimmy Ables,* he titled his book, writing it now on his computer, which he'd set up across the room from his own altar, a china cabinet filled with memorabilia. On the wall next to it, hung an enlargement of a black-and-white photo he'd taken of his Martita when she was thirty-two. Mami's face filled the frame; her gaze followed him around the room and through all the journeys he detailed in his book. He finished it a year later and printed twelve original copies. He had each professionally bound, gifting Ani and me and the family with near to 500 pages containing the stories from his heart.

To me, this inheritance is worth so much more than money.

• • •

Daddy and I had established a ritual a few years before Mami died. Each day, I'd call him at 5:30 p.m. to get an update on my mother's condition. Our talks also provided him with a way to vent his feelings, something he did in a roundabout way. He was, after all, a man of his era, one who'd learned at an early age to keep his feelings checked and to himself. He believed that a strong man was a silent one where emotions were concerned. When I called, he'd pick up on the first ring. I'd say, "How are you, Daddy?" and no matter what kind of day he'd had, his reply was the same: "I'm sitting on a cloud, honey, with my feet hanging down."

I quickly came to depend on our daily chats. Most times I was in the middle of writing a book set in El Salvador or Mexico, and I usually had questions about topography, weather, farm crops, the military, the guerrilla, armaments, the government, etc., etc., and so forth. Daddy was my personal encyclopedia. I'd ask, he'd answer. I have pads filled with notes I collected during our conversations.

And he confessed that he, too, looked forward to the end of the day, to his martini and the phone ringing. Over time, he began to open up about himself. Sometimes, when I asked how he was feeling, he'd say, "Estoy triste, honey. Triste triste." I'm sad. Sad, sad.

When Jim and I were living in San Diego that spring of 2001, Daddy began complaining about an itch. It was driving him crazy, he said. His arms itched; his back itched; the area around his waist itched. Fabric softener came immediately to mind. Ani's housekeeper was especially fond of those scented squares that went into the drier. In fact, I myself was so sensitive to them that I began to buy the perfume-free kind. I spoke to my sister about this and it was agreed that they would do the same.

But Daddy's itching continued. Soon, the dizzy spells commenced. This followed with bouts of nausea.

When he walked, he lost his balance and had to steady himself on things. Naturally, inner-ear trouble was suspected. Labrynthitis and Ménière's disease to be exact. Visits to specialists ensued. Tests given, which did not prove or disprove our suspicions. Though drugs were prescribed to ease his alarming discomforts, Daddy's maladies escalated. The nausea became so severe that he'd vomit two or three times an hour. Dehydration was a constant threat and on two occasions he had to be rushed to the emergency room for IV fluids. In addition, Daddy's balance was affected, so much so that at times he'd crumple to the floor.

All these troubles I monitored over the phone in long talks with my sister. When I spoke each day with Daddy, he would not dwell on how he felt, but turned our conversation to other topics, the most relevant of which was that my third novel, *The Weight of All Things,* was published and there were reviews and articles about it to discuss.

When my book tour brought me to Miami in early April, I brought with me a few motion sickness bracelets, hoping these might ease Daddy's dizziness and nausea. These provided a remedy for seafaring travelers; they consisted of a wide band of stretchy fabric with a round magnet attached. The magnet was positioned over a pressure point on the wrist, thus providing acupressure to the area responsible for balance. I placed one on each of Daddy's wrists. We raised a prayer to Our Holy Mother for help.

But the bracelets provided no relief. We turned then to the possibility of a stroke, an aneurysm, a brain tumor, so CAT scans, MRIs and MRAs were prescribed. When results came in, all these possibilities were discarded.

In late June, Daddy's nightmare began to include insomnia. On July 4th, I flew to Miami to help my sister and keep my father company. He was being hospitalized for the third time, again with severe dehydration. More tests were performed. He suffered them all, returning to his room where he spent the day propped against pillows, his eyes closed to forestall the nausea and dizziness.

To help him pass the time, I read aloud from his favorite books about the Civil War. In particular, he wanted to hear about Chamberlain's advance across Gravelly Run. I read these passages over and over for him. We discussed *Night of the Radishes,* the novel I was starting to write. Part of the book is set in Oaxaca, Mexico, and early on I had envisioned a subplot involving drug growing in the Chiapas area. Daddy returned there in his mind, describing the area and the best places for marijuana and poppies to thrive. (This subplot I ultimately rejected.)

Daddy was hospitalized for ten days in which all the tests he was given proved inconclusive. And so the hospital released him to a rehabilitation facility, for his symptoms had grown graver: in addition to the vomiting, his speech had become slurred; he began to lose his motor coordination. He could not walk. He could not feed himself.

Ani and I. We are Latino sisters and in our Latino family it is inconceivable, unless absolutely necessary, to place a loved one in a "facility" away from home. Daddy had his suite waiting for him. He had his altar containing his cherished memories; he had Mami's big photo looking down on him in consolation. At home, he also had Carlos Emilio, his very own private doctor, and

Carlos Emilio's colleagues, all of them very fond of don Jimmy, and always willing to make trips to the house for consultation.

But despite these comforts, Daddy's conditioned worsened. After four days of trying to handle him alone, Ani and I realized that we did not have the physical strength to lift him from bed, nor hold him up on trips to the bathroom. We hired two male nurses who came to the house in 12-hour shifts. It took a while for Daddy to adjust to the fact that he needed this kind of help, but he soon did.

I stayed on at my father's side, watching with a breaking heart his steady decline. The most distressing was to hear the way his mind was being affected: what he said did not make sense. We asked him to write down his thoughts, but this resulted in a page of zigs and dots and long lines. Sometimes you could make out the shadow of a word: "strong," "beautiful," "sense." He had frequent hallucinations, and was restless and agitated. At times, he turned violent, a terrible thing to see in a pacific man.

Carlos Emilio became convinced that Daddy's condition was related to some kind of problem in the cerebellum, the seat of motor coordination and of the messages sent from the brain to the mouth as speech. It wasn't that Daddy couldn't think. He understood what was said to him and responded by nodding or shaking his head, but what he could not do was to think something and then communicate what he thought.

My personal encyclopedia was being shelved for good.

At the end of our collective ropes, Carlos Emilio asked a friend, a neurologist, to visit and examine Daddy and give us an opinion.

This generous, merciful doctor arrived on a Sunday afternoon. We sat in the living room and he listened to our full story. He examined the films we'd gathered from all the tests. He went into Daddy's room and performed a thorough manual examination of Daddy's arms, legs, feet, eyes. He asked questions, listened closely to the attempted responses. When he was satisfied, the doctor patted Daddy's hand. "Duermase, don Jimmy." Go to sleep, don Jimmy.

The news was devastating. Horrifying, actually. Daddy had a Prion disease called Gertmann, Strussler, Sheinker.

"La vaca loca," the doctor said. Mad cow disease.

The human form of mad cow disease (bovine spongiform encephalopholy) is called Cruetzfeld Jacob disease. Daddy's condition was a rare form of it. It was fatal. At most, he had six months to live.

At the news, I think I might have gone a little mad myself. I know it took all my strength not to throw open Ani's front door and go screaming down the street. Instead, and later that afternoon, when I was sitting with Daddy and he asked what the doctor had discovered, I had to tell the truth. But I told it in a veiled sort of way.

"He said you're very sick, Daddy."

Daddy nodded, his pale blue eyes glistening.

I swallowed hard and continued, "Remember the many times you've told me how you're ready to be with Mami?"

Another nod.

"Well, I think you're on that road, Daddy. It's all up to God, but I think that soon you'll be with your Martita again."

This time, one tear slipped past Daddy's eyelid and slowly slid down his cheek.

I pulled him close. I buried my head against my Daddy Chulo's chest lest he see the depth of my sorrow.

• • •

In August, I had to leave Miami to return home and get ready for my teaching stint at Bread Loaf in Vermont. I had thought of canceling, but truth is, the money would come in handy. Daddy's care was costing two hundred and fifty dollars a day. I said "so long" while he was sitting up in his big chair, Mami's photo looking on. To think of that leave-taking now is so painful that I don't have the strength to fully describe it. I did, of course, tell my father where I was going and when I'd be back, for I planned to return just after Bread Loaf. But what makes it all so wrenching now, is that I never saw my father alive again. I was on the airplane returning to him, Susana's urn on my lap, when he passed away an hour before we landed in Miami.

• • •

Those ten days at Bread Loaf were made lighter because I'd been given a chance to make things right again. I returned to an approachable, generous faculty. I returned to smiling participants, writers who felt lifted up, who understood that to be present on campus was a reward in and of itself. In my own workshop, I was pleased to work with writers who, though they might not have been ready to be published, were willing to work hard to make their dreams come true.

As was the custom at Bread Loaf, all faculty members did a reading. Readings were the highlight of the day. They occurred in the big barn converted into the Little Theater, behind the same podium at which John Irving and Robert Stone and Tim O'Brien had read way back in '83. Back when I was a cowering writer with dreams in my heart. A writer with a heart bruised by an unkind writer's cutting remarks.

Stepping up to that podium, I began my reading by *not* reading, but by telling a story. I told the story of my experience at Bread Loaf ten years earlier. I didn't hold back. I recounted every single detail. I ended by exhorting all those eager writers in the audience to not give up. To stay the course. Believe in yourselves, I said. Believe in yourselves despite a sea of criticism. Be tenacious. Keep faith with the page. Write with your heart, especially when your heart is breaking.

At Bread Loaf, mine certainly was.

• • •

Daddy died one week before September 11th. Susana's urn was buried with him. In my studio, as I prepared the urn for my trip back to Miami, I'd unscrewed the bolts that held the top on the urn and extracted a handful of her remains to place on my own personal altar. Sitting here now, at my computer, I lift my eyes and there she is. If I look higher, past the sliding glass door of my studio, up above the trees, a bank of clouds drift by. Perched on the cloud are Mami and Daddy with their Susanita. The three of them hold hands. Their feet are hanging down.

• • •

The ensuing year proved to be an emotional catastrophe. I'd never suffered from depression before, but after I returned from Daddy's funeral, my personal grief entwined with our national grief over what had befallen our country and I fell into a hole so deep that getting out of bed seemed almost unfathomable. When I did manage to rise, I'd remain in my nightgown and robe, for it was too much of a chore to change into day clothes when soon I'd be needing those night clothes again. Unbeknownst to Jim, I spent a great deal of time in my studio walk-in closet. It is a roomy closet and built on an interior wall so that when you close the door, the space goes pitch black. I dragged cushions in there to sit on and rest my head against. I brought in my rosary, though trying to pray was near to impossible. I'd kept one of Daddy's books about the Civil War, a book that had especially sustained him after Mami's death. I brought that book into the closet with me, knowing that on its pages Daddy's tears had fallen.

I pressed that book so tightly to my heart.

I was under contract to my publisher for *Night of the Radishes* and I hadn't written a single word and my deadline was less than a year away. After a time, I forced myself to leave the closet and sit at my computer. I wrote that book in nine months. Is it any wonder that the novel is all about depression? About an identical twin who loses her twin sister, her mother and her father? About the emotional malignancy of keeping secrets?

• • •

Thanks to time, Zoloft, prayers, the support of my family and friends, my depression lifted after I finished the novel. The saving grace of stories—writing *Night of the Radishes* certainly proved their power. In 2002, for Christmas, Jim and I flew to Oaxaca, Mexico, for the holidays and for *la noche de los rábanos,* the Night of the Radishes festival. I had seen it once before, but Jim hadn't. My novel featured this festival and I wanted Jim to experience it.

The festival takes place on December 23rd and has been celebrated every year since it began in 1898. The radishes are giant, inedible tubers grown especially for carving into tableaux. The carvings are exhibited in booths set around the town square. The scenes that year included mariachi bands, troupes of dancers, the Holy Family, the Baby Jesus in his crèche, farm animals and angels, a variety of incarnations of the Virgin Mary, and an assortment of Saints, each in fancy robes. All created from radishes. From radish skins—bright red, pink, blush. From radish flesh and radish tops. All made by carving pieces and sometimes joining them together with toothpicks serving as tiny dowels.

The festival was extraordinary that year. Hundreds and hundreds of people milled around the square and its surrounding streets, enjoying the mild night, the food in the stands, the radish displays, and each other. The winning carving featured a colonial church (carved facade, towers, bells), fronting a bricked plaza, graced by an entire crèche scene. The talented, lucky family who carved it came away with $1,000 dollars (*not* pesos!), a veritable fortune for an Oaxacan artisan.

Before returning home, I decided to do something I'd been wanting to do each time I visited Oaxaca. I signed up for a *temazcal,* a healing ritual much like the Native American sweat lodge ceremony. The word comes from the Nahuatl, the language of the Aztecs, and means "bath" and "home." Mariana Arroyo Cabrera, whose family owns Las Bugambilias Bed and Breakfast in town, offers this purifying herbal bath in her country home.

I took a taxi up there, and soon was walking through her gate, into a garden abloom with color and scent. As directed, I took the path that led to the back, to a small adobe building where the *temazcalera's* cleansing ceremony would take place. The path meandered under a wide arbor spilling vines, past flower and herb beds. I felt like Dorothy, walking down the yellow brick road.

When I reached the little building, I stepped into tranquility. Swathed floor to ceiling with vaporous drapes, the entire room was a church of sorts. Set against one wall were wooden columns topped with capitals on which rested lighted candles and statues of old santos. In the center of the wall, worm-eaten pedestals rose to frame a large gilded image of Jesus and His Sacred Heart. Soft angelic music emanating from somewhere lent an air of reverence to the room. And everywhere there was the scent of flowers and herbs, an aromatic heaven.

Before the ritual, as Mariana suggested, I took time to center myself while sitting on one of the large pillows before the Heart of Jesus. Soon, she came out to tend to me herself. She was barefoot and dressed in an indigenous long *huipil,* her head wrapped in colorful textiles and adorned with ribbons. She showed me to a small dressing room where I disrobed and wrapped myself loosely in the large cotton sheet she provided. She escorted me to the *temazcal.* Everything about her, her voice, her touch, her stride, was quietly reassuring.

To enter the bath chamber we each crawled through

a small door. A single candle dimly lit the inside, a space tall and wide enough for both of us. I sat cross-legged on the hot adobe floor; she knelt in the corner beside a mound of heated volcanic rocks, much like you find in saunas. Here, the rocks were overlaid with boughs of rosemary and lavender and eucalyptus. Mariana commenced to chant in an indigenous tongue. She sent a spray of water over the rocks and the medicinals, and quickly the room steamed up. Soon, I was sweating heavily, the very purpose of the bath. I felt my pores open up and in minutes my sheet and I were soaked through. My scalp, my hair, my face dripped water. Breathe deeply, she said, and I pulled in the fragrant, hot air, allowed it to fill my head, my chest.

After some time, she took up rosemary branches that she'd bundled into a broom and began to sweep me clean. A *limpia* it is called, a cleansing. She drummed my head gently with the scented branches. Down and over they went, over my soaked body. Down and away. Prickly and aromatic. Each beat, each stroke was accented by her lyrical chants, and although what she intoned was foreign to me, my heart understood every syllable and phrase. Be cleansed, she was saying. Be cleansed of past preoccupations. Be freed of old unreachable expectations.

She stepped outside for a while so that I might meditate. At my request, she took the candle with her, pulled the little door closed so that I remained in the moist hot darkness, which was as comforting as my mother's womb.

I dropped the sheet away from me. Sitting on the floor, my legs stretched out, I leaned back against the wall and wept.

I wept with sorrow, my life fluttering behind my eyes much like images on a screen. Time to let go. Of perfectionism, of that hypersensitivity that had helped turn my gut to mush. Time to surrender. Surrender the guilt I felt about divorce. About leaving my children. The guilt I felt about having survived while Susana, my baby sister, had not. The grief and guilt that had toppled me at not having been at my Daddy's side when he flew up into Mami's arms.

And I wept with gratitude for all the good things that had come into my life. Good parents, now both dead. My darling sisters, one gone, one thankfully not. Marvelous, understanding sons. A beloved husband. Devoted friends. Though late to come, a writing career that had opened up my world.

I gave special thanks to my own constitution, which had withstood a grand emotional assault and had not reverted into illness again.

When Mariana crawled back into the chamber, she rinsed me clean. She used rosewater to do it. An entire pail of rosewater, which she slowly poured over my head.

• • •

Each year, on October 26, the anniversary of my surgery, I write a little note to my spout. I use a permanent marker and the sheet of purple plastic that was wrapped around a bouquet I received at the hospital. Ritualistically, I lay this sheet down beside me when I'm about to change my bag. Upon it go the supplies in my kit. Each week, when I change my bag, the yearly notes I've written are there to greet me.

"Thank you, thank you. You're an incredible helper. I'm so glad I have you."

"Still the best little spout in the world. I thank you so much."

"Thank you for your great and loyal work, for all you do to keep me healthy."

There are seven more notes written on the sheet, not any of them great literature, but each written with all my love to what has become a best friend.

Which brings me to the question: Our stoma, friend or foe?

As for me, I opt for friendship.

My stoma, my bag and me.

We are the best of buddies.

EPILOGUE

I SIT IN MY ROCKING CHAIR, that ancient red one where I once nursed my babies and sang to them. I am holding Harper Henry Title, my first grandchild, the son of my son, Chris, and his wife, Karen. I've waited so long for this. I am 64 and I now have a child in my arms once more. A child whose blood is my blood, a child who looks so much like his father that it's like I'm holding baby Chris all over again.

When Harper was born, and minutes later, pink and healthy and squealing with life, he was laid under the warmer-lamp of the cleanup table, my heart bloomed with joy. A few hours later, when I watched my ex, his grandfather, cautiously approach Harper's crib to meet him, my ex-husband bent his head and wept.

Dear God, I said to myself, noting this. All is forgiven. I forgive him. I forgive myself.

Now, with me in the rocker, Harper looks up into my face, his expression intense and sober. I believe he can see the woman I once was, the woman I've worked hard to become. Harper's tiny fingers are wrapped around my finger and make a circle.

Life is a circle, a spiral of blessings. The blessing of my grandson's presence is something that feels very much like redemption.

I sing softly to my boy, that old song I used to sing to Chris and Jon, *Where are you going, my little one, little one?*

Harper narrows his eyes, tightens his grip around my finger.

With all my love, I smile at him.

I know who I am.

I am a bag lady, a woman healed.

By the grace of God, I am a grateful woman saved.

And I know where I've been.

I know where I'm going.

Joyfully, I stride into the world, my own true stories restoring and preserving me.

ADDITIONAL HELPFUL INFORMATION

BOOK SALES AND SPEAKING ENGAGEMENTS

bag lady: A Memoir has not as yet been released for national distribution through the usual retail channels. However, until it is, copies are available through our website: **www.sandrabenitez.com.** All major credit cards are accepted.

QUANTITY DISCOUNTS for bulk purchases are available to medical and nursing organizations, hospitals, health care insurers and medical products manufacturers. For details, email us at **benitezbooks@msn.com** or call Jim Kondrick at **952-933-1657.**

COMPLIMENTARY COPIES will be furnished to medical and health care publications wishing to review the book. See the email and phone information above.

To inquire about Sandra Benítez's fees and availability for a speaking engagement at your event, email Sandra at **benitezbooks@msn.com.**

MY KIT AND ITS CONTENTS

Everyone's kit will be different, of course. But this is what works for me.

I selected a small make-up bag. There are many to be found. Mine has a zipper, is compact, waterproof and holds all my supplies and fits nicely in my purse.

In it I keep the items I use on a weekly basis and other items I might use if the need arises. As the items are used, I replace them immediately so that my kit is always "ready to go!"

• • •

2 appliances. I use ConvaTec Active Life, a one-piece drainable pouch with the Stomahesive Skin Barrier.

12 or so non-sterile gauze wipes for cleaning the skin around my stoma. Any brand will do. I wet a few with warm water for wiping and then a few dry ones for patting my skin dry.

1 small bottle of Nexcare No Sting Liquid Bandage Spray. You can get this at Walgreens. This spray is a miracle because it doesn't sting! After my skin is clean and dry, I spray the area that will be covered by the appliance to set down a waterproof barrier. I allow it to dry before continuing.

1 tube of ConvaTec Stomahesive Paste. In case I need extra barrier protection. Most times I do not.

2 Hefty Scrap Bags. In your grocery's disposable-bags aisle! They come 50 bags to the box. These are fabulous for disposing of old bag, soiled wipes, etc. The Hefty bags are white so there is no visual information when tossing them. Each comes with a Tear-Off tie that can be used for secure disposal.

Roll of Curad Wet-Pruf adhesive tape. To mend leaking-emergencies.

1 Sharpie, fine-point, permanent marker. Mine is green! I write the day I change my bag on the top of the webbed circle that's adhered to my tummy. The Sharpie is waterproof, so date won't fade in the shower.

This is just me, but I keep a holy card of the Virgin Mary in my kit. It's nice to see her there each time I open my kit.

LIST OF USEFUL ORGANIZATIONS

Crohn's and Colitis Foundation
of America (CCFA)
386 Park Avenue South, 17th Floor
New York, NY 10016
1-800-932-2423
www.ccfa.org

United Ostomy Associations of America, Inc.
(UOAA)
19772 MacArthur Blvd., Suite 200
Irvine, CA 92612-2405
1-800-826-0826
www.uoaa.org

American Cancer Society
1-800-227-2345
www.cancer.org

ConvaTec, Inc.
PO Box 5254
Princeton, NJ 08543
1-800-422-8811
www.convatec.com

(Other appliance manufacturers include: Coloplast, Inc. 1-800-533-0464, Hollister, Inc. 1-800-323-4060, and Nu-Hope, Inc. 1-800-899-5017)

LIST OF INFORMATIVE BOOKS

Barbara Barrie. *Don't Die of Embarrassment: Life After Colostomy and Other Adventures.* New York, NY: Scribner. 1999.

Rolf Benirschke, with Mike Yorkey. *Alive & Kicking: The True Story of an NFL star's battle with ulcerative colitis, ostomy surgery and hepatitis C.* San Diego, CA. Rolf Benirschke Enterprises, Inc. 1996.

Barbara Dorr Mullen, Kerry Anne McGinn, RN, BSN, OCN. *The Ostomy Book: Living Comfortably With Colostomies, Ileostomies and Urostomies.* Boulder, CO: Bull Publishing Company. 1992.

Fred Saibil, MD. *Crohn's Disease & Ulcerative Colitis: Everything You Need to Know.* Buffalo, NY: Firefly Books. 1996.

Dr. Craig A. White. *Positive Options for Living with Your Ostomy.* Alameda, CA: Hunter House, Inc. Publishers. 2002.

Jon Zonderman and Ronald S. Vender, M.D. *Understanding Crohn's Disease and Ulcerative Colitis.* Jackson, MS: University Press of Mississippi. 2000.

OTHER

Blue Wave Relaxation, Stress Relief Training
Peg Evans, MS, info@bluewaverelax.com, 305-899-9943
I heartily recommend her *Blue Wave Relaxation* CD.